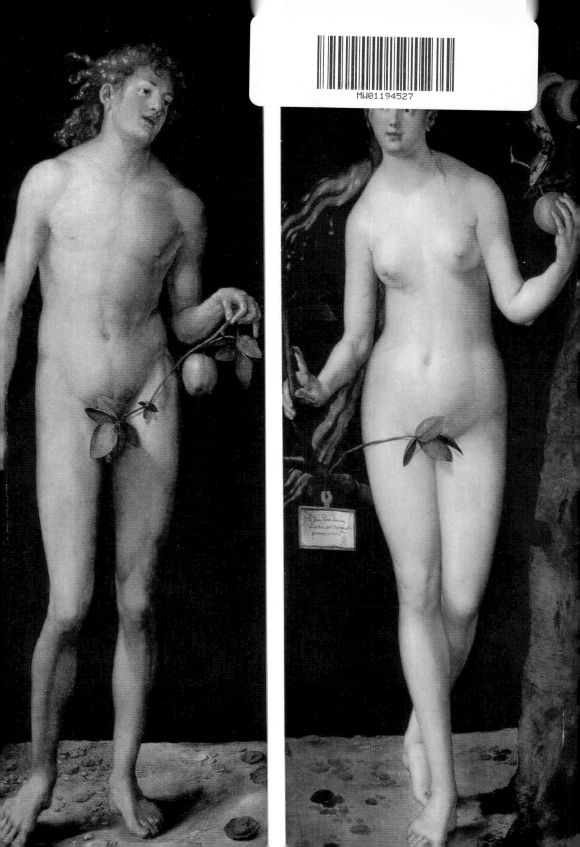

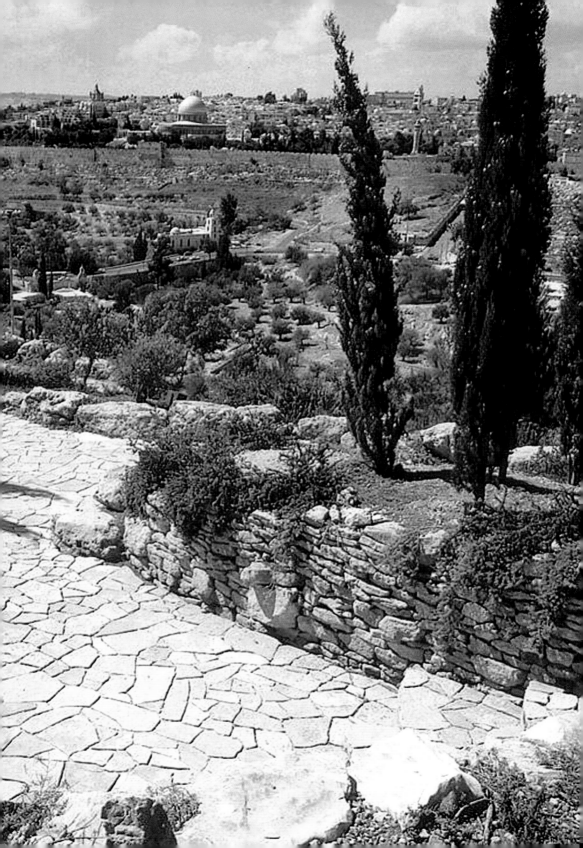

Healing Herbs of the Holy Land

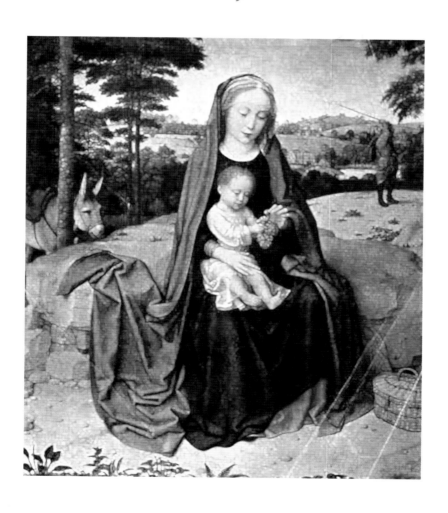

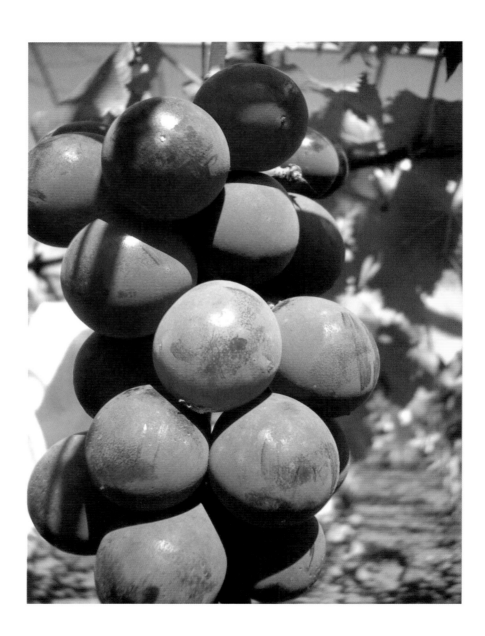

Healing Herbs of the Holy Land

Herbs from the Bible for Today

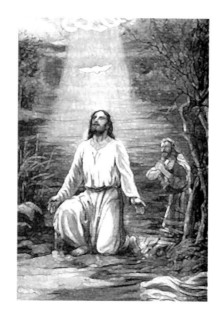

Dan Wolf

Astrolog Publishing House Ltd.

Cover Design: Daniel Akerman
Language Consultants: Leora Hadas, Marion Duman
Layout and Graphics: Daniel Akerman
Production Manager: Dan Gold

P. O. Box 1123, Hod Hasharon 45111, Israel
Tel: 972-9-7412044
Fax: 972-9-7442714

© Astrolog Publishing House Ltd. 2004

ISBN 965-494-182-1

Published by Astrolog Publishing House 2004

*M*any years ago, I was a member of a research delegation in New Guinea, our objective being to find medicinal plants that could help cure diseases known as "tropical diseases". Our guide was a local doctor, and every conversation with him would begin with the sentence: "Remember, here you can learn how the ancient people, the first ones, lived... The tribes that live here eat the same food their forefathers ate, succumb to the same illnesses, and use the same medicines provided by nature..."

Years later, I reached the Near East, where I visited the Bedouin who live in Israel and Jordan. One of the elders of the tribe that was extending its hospitality to me said exactly the same thing: "We live in the same way as people lived here one, two thousand years ago... as in the days of the Prophet [Muhammed] and the days of your Jesus. We use the same plants for healing..."

Apparently, that was the moment the idea to write a book dedicated to the medicinal plants that have always been used in the land that is sacred to three religions – Judaism, Christianity and Islam – was born. In order to learn about the time of Jesus,

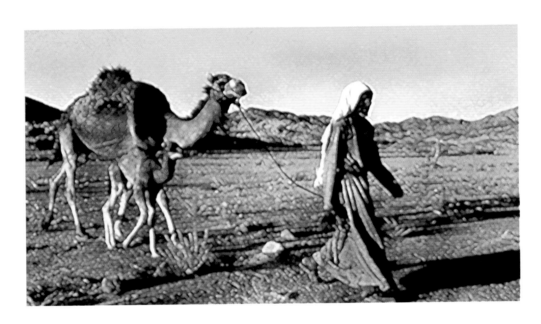

I explored the holy books (the Hebrew Bible and the New Testament) and learned how the plants had been used in that period. I subsequently conducted comprehensive research in order to identify the medicinal plants of biblical times against the names of the plants that are common today, and I found out which of the plants are still used. Finally, I investigated the uses of the plants today.

The result is this colorful book, which presents some forty plants that were used during the time of Jesus and are in use to this day for medicinal purposes, cures, and healing. The book is actually a guide that enables 21st-century people to visit the Holy Land where Jesus lived and make use of the knowledge that accumulated there…

The book proves that "there's nothing new under the sun", because today, in the Holy Land, the herbs and medicinal plants are still used for their healing properties, exactly as they were during the times of Moses, Jesus and Muhammed!

Dan Wolff

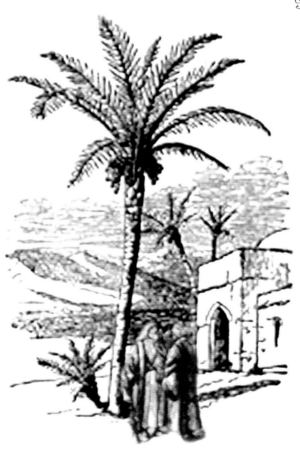

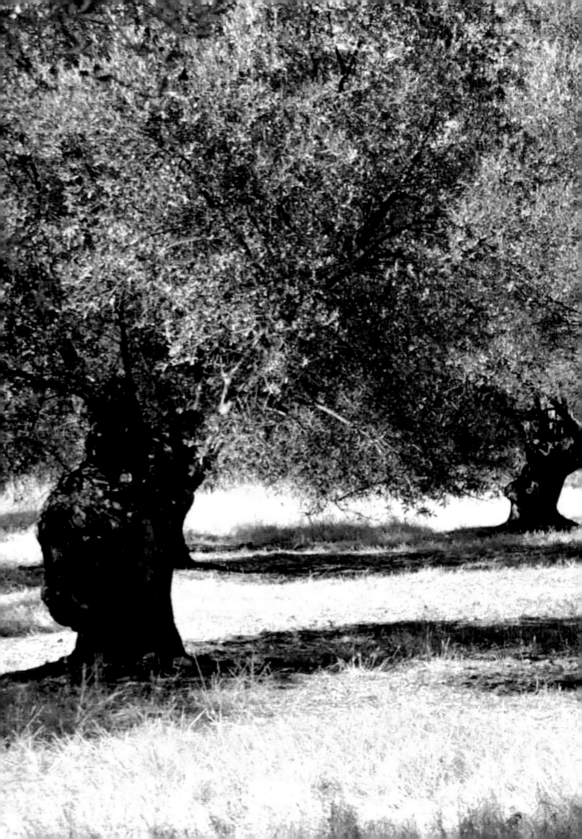

Contents

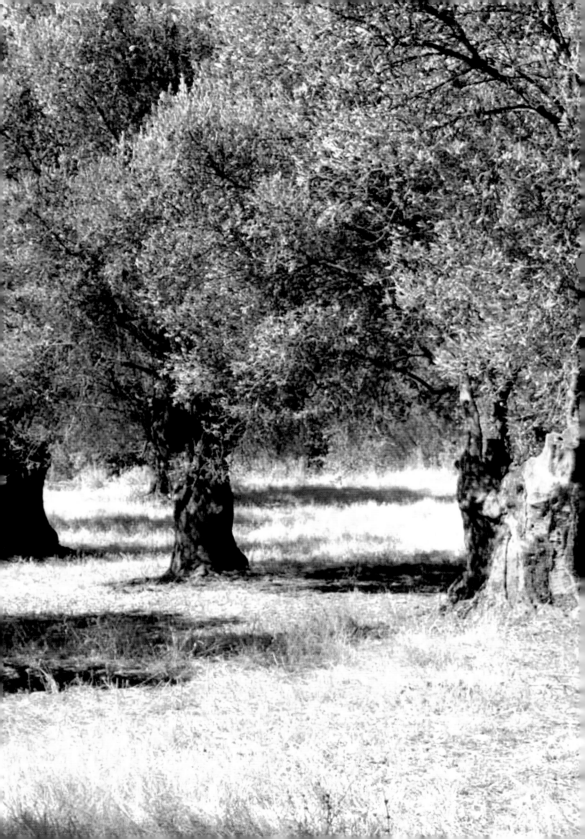

Almond

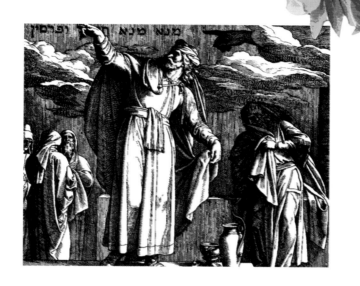

"Moreover the word of the Lord came unto me, saying, Jeremiah, what seest thou? And I said, I see a rod of an almond tree."

Jeremiah 1:11

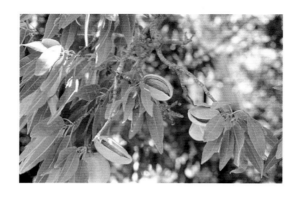

"And their father Israel said unto them, If it must be so now, do this; take of the best fruits in the land in your vessels, and carry down the man a present, a little balm, and a little honey, spices, and myrrh, nuts, and Almonds."

Genesis 43:11

"And it came to pass, that on the morrow Moses went into the tabernacle of witness; and, behold, the rod of Aaron for the house of Levi was budded, and brought forth buds, and bloomed blossoms, and yielded Almonds."

Numbers 17:8

M ore than any other, this tree is a symbol of spring renewal. While all the other trees still boast bare branches in the grip of winter, the almond tree blooms in beautiful pink or white flowers. In summer, these flowers grow into the familiar soft, elongated fruits, which were one of the more common and desired fruits of the Holy Land in ancient times. Children, especially, were often given this sweet treat.

The almond is still a favorite in Israeli kindergartens. According to the children's story, the almond's early-blooming flowers were created by a good fairy's kiss as a birthday gift to the tree. I remember celebrating the almond tree's birthday – the "New Year of the trees" – as a small child.

The almond is a useful medicinal plant, the oil of its fruits being the most effective part. Three spoonfuls of almond oil a day cure stomach-aches, dry coughs, intestinal parasites and lung diseases. Moreover, almond oil stimulates lactation in new mothers. Three drops of oil help to cure ear infections.

For skin diseases, four ounces of almonds can be ground into a powder that is then cooked in a quart of water for half an hour. A towel is dipped into the resulting mixture and rubbed on to the infected skin.

Finally, almonds have been known to increase the libido and gradually counteract impotence.

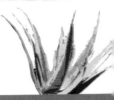

Aloe Vera

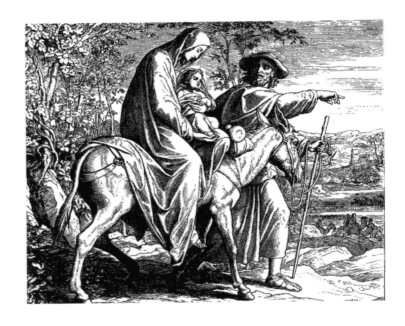

"All thy garments smell of myrrh, and aloes, and cassia, out of the ivory palaces, whereby they have made thee glad."

Psalms 45:8

"And there came also Nicodemus, which at the first came to Jesus by night, and brought a mixture of myrrh and aloes, about an hundred pound weight."

John 19:39

"I have perfumed my bed with myrrh, aloes, and cinnamon."

Proverbs 7:17

*L*ong renowned as a healing herb, the aloe vera is a two-foot-high, thick-stemmed bush with fleshy, sword-shaped bluish or grayish leaves with jagged edges. In the summer, thick clusters of yellow flowers bloom on its stems.

The main use of the aloe vera in ancient times was not for medicinal purposes, but rather for embalming. The Egyptians applied the juice of its fleshy leaves to wounds on corpses that were to be mummified in order to keep decay at bay and to serve as a kind of perfume. They believed that by doing so, the dead be healed prior to entering the afterlife.

Socrates was quoted as saying that anyone who grew the aloe vera in his garden would gain riches and prosperity. Alexander the Great took that advice and used it as a medication for his troops; the plant seemed to have worked just fine for him. The aloe vera is one of the oldest natural remedies in the world – as the ancient Greeks noted more than 2,000 years ago.

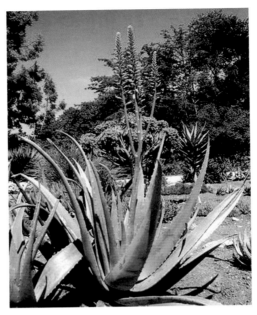

Modern medicine has made the aloe vera as renowned as it was in folk medicine for treating skin problems. When cut, the fleshy leaves exude a rust-colored gel that soothes and cools inflamed skin. When half a leaf oozing with gel is placed on burns, infections, stings, and dry skin, it works wonders. Massaging the stomach with that same gel, alleviates stomach-aches, particularly in children.

The gel of the aloe vera is also an efficient natural laxative. It can be drunk either as is, or mixed with an alcoholic beverage such as wine or whiskey. Finally, a few drops of the juice of squeezed aloe leaves can cure eye infections.

Apple

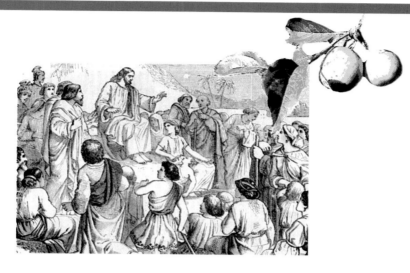

"The vine is dried up, and the fig tree languisheth; the pomegranate tree, the palm tree also, and the apple tree, even all the trees of the field, are withered: because joy is withered away from the sons of men."

Joel 1:12

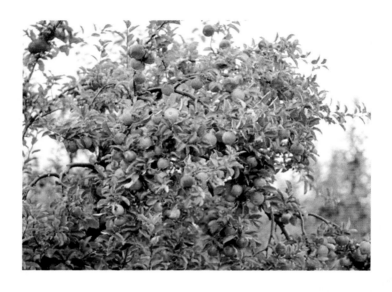

"As the apple tree among the trees of the wood, so is my beloved among the sons. I sat down under his shadow with great delight, and his fruit was sweet to my taste."

Song of Solomon 2:3

J doubt that most people today, enjoying this sweet fruit, are aware of its long history, its healing qualities, or its great symbolism. Apples were cultivated by the ancient Egyptians in the 13th century BCE and spread throughout the Mediterranean. Four thousand years ago, Persian soldiers stuck gold-coated apples on their spears, and cities were named after the tree.

The apple tree is about ten feet tall, and grows mostly in orchards nowadays. Its widespread branches are auburn-brown and covered in a thin fluff when the tree is young. Its leaves are shiny on the upper side and velvety on the lower side, their edges jagged. The flowers, which bloom in spring, emerge in pink-white clusters, giving the tree a festive look. The shape and color of the fruit, as we all know, differ according to the countless subspecies that have been cultivated.

Most famous, however, is the red apple, a symbol of health and love since ancient times. King Solomon wrote of it as a beautiful tree exuding a calming scent and compared a lovely maiden's breasts to its smooth roundness. According to the Song of Solomon, bright red apples were considered a cure for the infamous "lovesickness" that has plagued the young since Biblical times.

But apples are a cure not only for lovesickness, and modern medicine has proved what countless mothers have known all along: apples are rich in a variety of vitamins and minerals, which are vital for overall health. They make digestion more efficient and are good for liver function. Apple juice helps prevent colds, flu and stomach infections and helps relieve aching joints, constipation and liver and kidney problems. A glass of apple juice a day will make us all healthier.

Since many of the apple's best qualities are in its peel, it is advisable to eat the apples or squeeze them for juice as they are, without peeling them.

barley

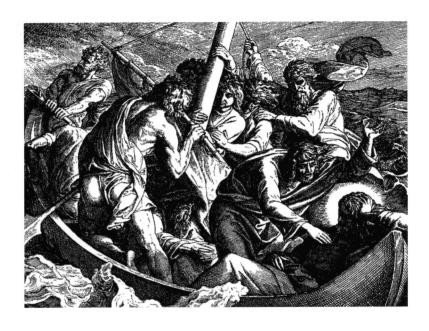

"There is a lad here, which hath five barley loaves and two small fishes: but what are they among so many?"

John 6:9

"And there came a man from Baal-shalisha, and brought the man of God bread of the firstfruits, twenty loaves of barley, and full ears of corn in the husk thereof. And he said, give unto the people, that they may eat."

II Kings 4:42

*B*arley may be a simple plant, but it has been vital to agriculture in the Middle East and all over the world since ancient times. It grows to a height of about two feet, with thin ears divided into threes growing along the stalk. Each ear blooms in a single small flower. The middle ear in the trio is the fertile one, which produces the grain used in making bread, beer, and countless other foods.

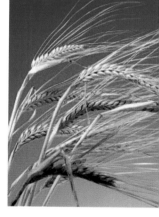

To treat urinary tract blockages and kidney stones, barley seeds should be boiled in water for an hour, filtered and drunk (four to five glasses a day). This is also a good remedy for nervousness and diabetes. Gargling with the mixture while still hot helps throat infections, and washing the eyes with it cleans and heals them.

Another way to exploit the barley's medicinal qualities is in a bath. A pound of seeds cooked in three quarts of water for an hour produce a medicinal bath that, in a half-hour soak, alleviates swelling in various parts of the body, and eases rashes and itching of the skin.

Castor-Oil Plant

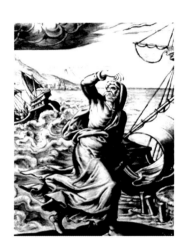

"And the Lord God prepared a gourd, and made it to come up over Jonah, that it might be a shadow over his head, to deliver him from his grief. So Jonah was exceeding glad of the gourd."

Jonah 4:6

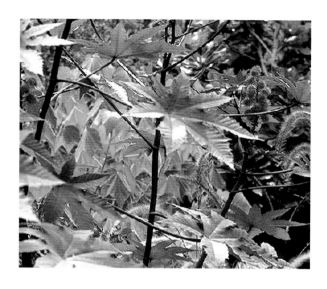

A highly poisonous but common bush, the castor-oil plant is tall – about 15 feet high – and peculiar. Its stems are hollow and of a curious reddish shade, as are its large star-shaped leaves. Its flowers grow in thick green clusters, and its fruits grow in the fall, containing pretty, spotted seeds. The oil extracted from the seeds is the only usable part of the plant – the rest is deadly.

The castor-oil plant has a curious property: it grows amazingly fast, and dies just as quickly if it lacks water. In both ancient and modern times, it became a metaphor for things that fall as quickly as they rise.

While the castor-oil plant became famous in the story of Jonah and his conversation with God after his encounter with the bush, few people are familiar with its botanical aspect. The castor-oil plant's harmless-looking seeds are, in fact, powerful hallucinogens…

The castor oil extracted from the plant's seeds may be notorious for its revolting taste, but its usefulness is indisputable. Traditional as well as modern medicine recognized its powers as a laxative. A spoonful of castor oil is as good as cure as there is for severe constipation and does wonders for an upset stomach, especially mixed with a spoonful of honey. Warmed, three drops of the oil can be applied to infected ears.

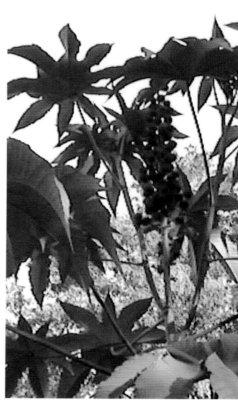

Rheumatic pains can also be treated with the oil by warming it and rubbing it into the aching joints. Warm castor oil is also used to open purulent wounds.

It must be noted that aside from all the medicinal qualities of castor oil, the rest of the plant, seeds and all, is extremely toxic. Only the oil may be used safely.

cinnamon

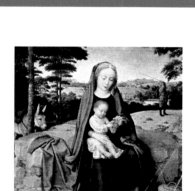

"I have perfumed my bed with myrrh, aloes, and cinnamon."

Proverbs 7:17

"Spikenard and saffron; calamus and cinnamon, with all trees of frankincense; myrrh and aloes, with all the chief spices."

Song of Solomon 4:14

"And cinnamon, and odours, and ointments, and frankincense, and wine, and oil, and fine flour, and wheat, and beasts, and sheep, and horses, and chariots, and slaves, and souls of men."

Revelation 18:13

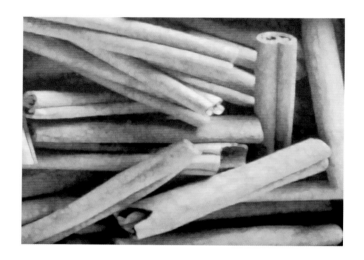

A well-known, familiar spice as well as a medicinal plant, cinnamon grows as a splendid evergreen tree, 50 feet in height. Its small egg-shaped leaves are dark on their upper side and light on their lower side, and exude a strong, pleasant scent. From May to December, it blooms in clusters of small yellow flowers with a silky surface. Its purple fruits grow all year round.

Cinnamon has been known for over five millennia, beginning, apparently, in China. It was a common plant and already a known spice in the Holy Land in Biblical times, as is evident in the Song of Songs. Nero, one of Rome's many crazy emperors, is said to have burned as much cinnamon as

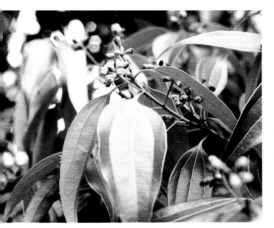

all the people of Rome used in a whole year at the funeral of his beloved wife. It is no wonder that he went on to burn other things.

In ancient times, cinnamon was used to cleanse the digestive tract, regulate menstrual periods, and even induce abortions. Today its qualities are recognized for treating coughs, colds, and even hiccups.

A teaspoonful of powdered cinnamon should be boiled in a glass of water, sweetened with honey and drunk. Mixed with pistachio resin, it relieves a sore throat and cures hoarseness.

In Morocco, ground cinnamon is mixed with lemon juice, spread on fabric, and tied around the head as a cure for headaches. Cinnamon tea is used to cleanse the kidneys and to cure impotence. In India, a mixture of cinnamon, black pepper and almonds is supposed to cure an upset stomach.

Common Olive

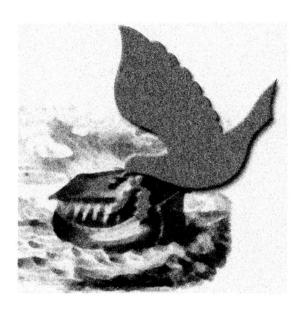

"*And the dove came in to him in the evening; and, lo, in her mouth was an olive leaf pluckt off: so Noah knew that the waters were abated from off the earth.*"

Genesis 8:11

"And for the entering of the oracle he made doors of olive tree: the lintel and side posts were fifth part of the wall. / The two doors also were of olive tree; and he carved upon them carvings of cherubims and palm trees and open flowers, and overlaid them with gold, and spread gold upon the cherubims, and upon the palm trees."

I Kings 6:31-32

"...Go forth unto the mount, and fetch olive branches, and pine branches, and myrtle branches, and palm banches, and branches of thick trees, to make booths, as it is written."

Nehemiah 8:15

"And thou shalt command the children of Israel, that they bring thee pure oil olive beaten for the light, to cause the lamp to burn always."

Exodus 27:20

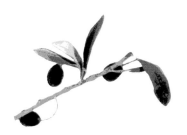

Perhaps the most familiar plant from the Bible and almost synonymous with the Holy Land, the common olive is a splendid evergreen tree that can reach a height of over 20 feet. Its powerful, extensive roots can penetrate solid stone, and its small leaves are dull green on the upper side and silvery-gray on the lower side. Its blossoms, which appear during the spring and early summer, in April and May, are small and white, and may bear fruit after its sixth year. This fruit comes in a green as well as a brown variety, if it is left to mature, and contains almost 50 percent oil. It

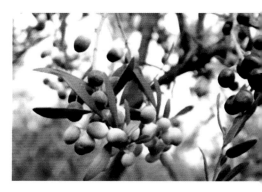

cannot be eaten straight off the tree since it contains a bitter substance that is extracted during the pressing process.

The common olive and its connection to the land of Israel has a rich history that dates back to the biblical period. According to the Bible, the Hebrews found olive trees when they first arrived in the Holy Land. Furthermore, the Scriptures relate how olive oil was exported to Egypt during the sixth century BCE. Olive pits were unearthed in archeological digs in several historical sites in Israel such as Megiddo and Beit She'an, which date back four millennia, while in the Galilee, thousand-year-old olive trees still exist today.

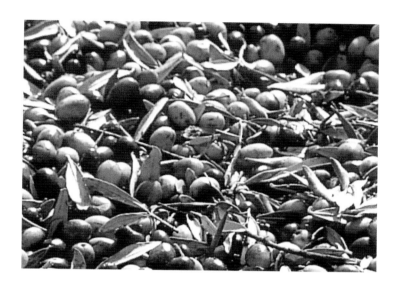

Because of the cultural, economic and religious importance of the olive tree, folklore and tales relating to it abound. According to legend, when King Solomon died, every tree in his garden bowed its head and shed its leaves, except for the olive, which remained upright and in full bloom. The trees, aghast, turned to the olive and asked: "Are you not ashamed? The wisest of men, who spoke the tongue of plants, is dead, yet you show no sign of grieving?" The olive sighed and replied: "You, my friends, must express your grief and bow down in mourning, but my sorrow is deeper. Behold my heart is consumed with it." Ever since, the heart of the olive tree, the interior of its trunk, is hollow. The same legend is told with regard to the destruction of the Temple.

The common olive has a great many medicinal uses. Its oil is most commonly used to help digestion. In addition, it has been proved to alleviate stomach pains, help get rid of kidney stones and abdominal parasites, and improve the appetite. In ancient times, wounds and burns were often treated with olive oil. It can be used to smooth and soften the skin, and it is effective in strengthening the roots of the hair. The heads of kings and prophets were anointed with olive oil for a reason…

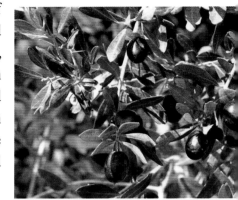

A spoonful of olive oil mixed with honey is a well-known remedy for relieving baby ailments such as coughs and respiratory diseases. Rubbing olive oil into aching joints alleviates the pain, while drops of olive oil mixed with vinegar can be used to treat ear infections. Boiling olives in water and drinking the resulting liquid can lower blood pressure and help diabetics. The olive is a marvelous plant that is effective against a vast array of human ailments and pains.

Cumin

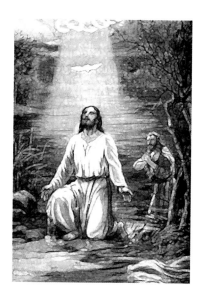

"When he hath made plain the face thereof, doth he not cast abroad the fitches, and scatter the cummin, and cast in the principal wheat and the appointed barley and the rie in their place?"

Isaiah 28:25

A popular spice since ancient times, cumin was put to a wide variety of uses all over the ancient East. It flavored fish and meat, it served as an appetizer, and, since time immemorial, was used in medicine. In ancient Rome, men would eat it in great quantities to give their faces an alabaster pallor, although how effective that method actually was is debatable.

In 13th- and 14th-century Europe, cumin was also a popular spice, and was believed to ensure love and prevent infidelity and adultery.

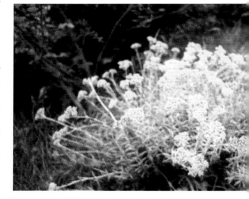

The cumin plant is about a foot high, with very thin, pale stems and blue-tinged leaves outspread in thin webs. The flowers, which bloom in the spring, come in pinkish-white umbels. The fruit of the cumin plant is elliptical and flat, sometimes covered in thin hairs.

Cumin seeds are good for speeding digestion and treating urinal blockages, liver diseases, breathing difficulties, and skin infections. A teaspoonful of seeds boiled in a cup of water is good for all stomach ailments. For rashes and skin diseases, boil two ounces of seeds in water for 20 minutes and gently spread the mixture on the infected skin.

In various places around the globe, cumin has a number of other uses, including the property of stanching nosebleeds among the Jews of Iraq.

Date Palm

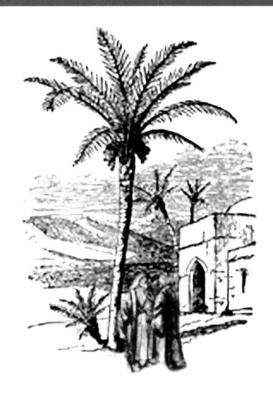

"The righteous shall flourish like the palm tree: he shall grow like a cedar in Lebanon."

Psalm 92:12

"The two doors also were of olive tree; and he carved upon them carvings of cherubims and palm trees and open flowers, and overlaid them with gold, and spread gold upon the cherubims, and upon the palm trees."

I Kings 6:32

"On the next day much people that were come to the feast, when they heard that Jesus was coming to Jerusalem, / Took branches of plam trees, and went forth to meet him, and cried, Hosanna: Blessed is the King of Israel that cometh in the name of the Lord."

John 12:12-13

"...Go forth unto the mount, and fetch olive branches, and pine branches, and myrtle branches, and palm banches, and branches of thick trees, to make booths, as it is written."

Nehemiah 8:15

"And ye shall take you on the first day the boughs of goodly trees, branches of palm trees, and the boughs of thick trees, and willows of the brook; and ye shall rejoice before the Lord your God seven days."

Leviticus 23:40

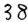

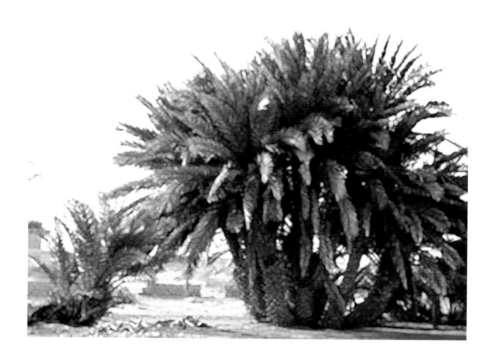

*T*he palm, which is yet another famous Holy Land plant, is an impressive tree that bears a sweet, luscious fruit. It is a very tall tree – frequently reaching a height of 60 feet – with a rough, ragged trunk devoid of branches. The large, stiff leaves whose shape gave the palm tree its name grow right at the top. The tree bears its fruit in huge clusters between August and December.

The scene of an oasis surrounded by palm trees is a familiar one. This tree does, in fact, thrive in the heart of the desert, unaffected by the harsh environment. For this reason, it became a symbol of prosperity and resilience, and even a metaphor for feminine beauty. Its fruit was an important food during the Hebrews' journey to the Holy Land, and is still a cherished symbol for the Jews. The thatch that is placed on top of the sukkot [booths] are made of date palm fronds as a reminder of the journey.

The dates that grow on the palm are very sweet and plentiful. Honey, sugar and a delicious juice are frequently extracted from them, and they can be eaten dried. Even today, palm leaves are woven into baskets and mats among by the Bedouins and other desert-dwellers, and its wood can be made into excellent furniture and, ironically enough, boats.

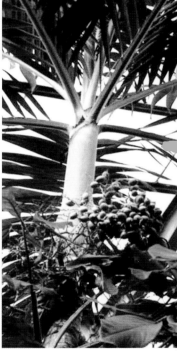

Dates serve as mild laxatives and are good for a myriad of digestive diseases, as well as being a good, satisfying food in cases of sudden hunger attacks. They are filling but not heavy. Dates are recommended for people who suffer from anemia as well as for blood donors.

Dates are also used for increasing men's vitality and sexual prowess. The date palm alleviates the symptoms of many venereal diseases: the patient bathes in a mixture of date pollen and hot water: a handful of pollen per quart of water. Roasted and ground palm seeds are effective when applied to open wounds.

Dill

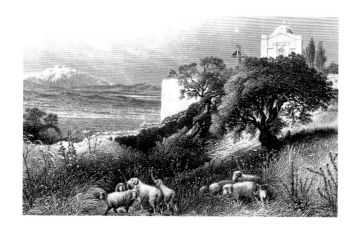

"Dill is not threshed with a threshing sledge, nor is a cart wheel rolled over cumin; but dill is beaten out with a stick, and cumin with a rod."

Isaiah 28:27

A herb as well as medicinal plant, dill is a herb of between two and four feet in height, with slender, hollow branched stems and feathery leaves. The flower is shaped like a yellow-white umbel and produces numerous bitter-tasting tiny seeds in the fall. The dill is an aromatic plant, all of whose parts produce a scent like much that of cumin.

As early as the Middle Ages, dill is mentioned as having been used for pickling – hence dill pickles – and was apparently used for this purpose much earlier on. Although it originated in Europe, it was a well-known herb in ancient Egypt, and was cultivated in the Holy Land.

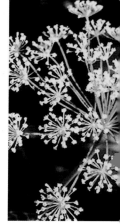

In the Middle Ages, dill had another important use: it was one of the key ingredients in many a wizard's spell and many a superstitious witch-hunter's arsenal.

The part of the dill that is primarily used in medicine is its seeds. Five teaspoonfuls of them boiled in water for 15 minutes serve as a cure for flatulence and stomach-aches. It is generally good for keeping the digestive tract healthy. Gargling with the mixture after breakfast and before bed prevents halitosis. A different quantity – one teaspoon of seeds rather than five – makes a remedy for eye infections.

Sweetening the drink with honey is recommended both for improving its taste and reinforcing its qualities.

European Box Thorn

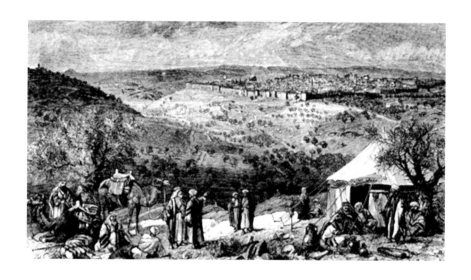

"I will plant in the wilderness the cedar, the shittah tree, and the myrtle, and the oil tree; I will set in the desert the fir tree, and the pine, and the box tree together."

Isaiah 41:19

J n the Bible, this thorny bush is not held in high regard. This is understandable, since it is not a friendly plant; it grows at the edges of fields, stubbornly refusing to be uprooted. In late summer, when it it is dry and leafless, it catches fire easily, thus endangering the adjacent orchards and fields. Despite its long thorns, however, it is not without its uses. To this today, it serves a good natural fence .

The box thorn is a three-foot-high bush with long arching branches and fleshy leaves. Its short thorns emerge from clusters of the leaves. It is not entirely devoid of beauty – in spring, it blooms in pink flowers that have a delicate, pleasant smell. The Bedouin in the Negev – especially young women – use the juice from the leaves for making tattoos, so the thorny bush engenders beauty as well.

The Bedouin have quite a few other uses for the box thorn, including the treatment of headaches, eye infections, stomach-aches and so on. An infusion made from a handful of the leaves boiled in water relieves stomach-aches and flatulence. The liquid can also be applied externally to irritated skin, scabies and eczema.

Boil about two teaspoonfuls of the box thorn's roots for ten minutes and drink four or five glasses of the filtrate in

Fig

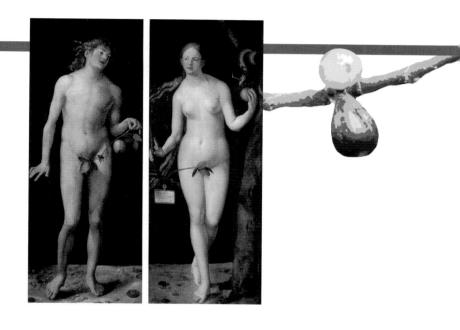

"And the eyes of them both were opened, and they knew that they were naked; and they sewed fig leaves together, and made themselves aprons."

Genesis 3:7

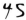

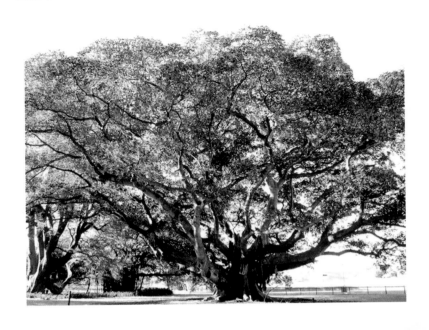

"And they came unto the brook of Eshcol, and cut down from thence a branch with one cluster of grapes, and they bare it between two upon a staff; and they brought of the pomegranates, and of the figs."

Numbers 13:23

"And Judah and Israel dwelt safely, every man under his vine and under his fig tree, from Dan even to Beer-sheba, all the days of Solomon."

I Kings 4:25

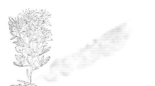

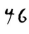

46

"And seeing a fig tree afar off having leaves, he came, if haply he might find any thing thereon: and when he came to it, he found nothing but leaves; for the time of figs was not yet."

Mark 11:13

"The fig tree putteth forth her green figs, and the vines with the tender grape give a good smell. Arise, my love, my fair one, and come away."

Song of Solomon 2:13

A tall tree with a thick trunk, the fig has large, rough-textured leaves shaped vaguely like a hand. It blooms in the spring, around March, with small ball-like flowers that may remain in full bloom until the fall. The fig bears fruit three times a year. The round fruit, which has a high sugar content, is picked between July and December.

The fig is found all over Israel, and has apparently existed there since the end of the Stone Age at least 8,000 years ago. It is said that the spies sent by Joshua to scout the Holy Land returned bearing figs.

Figs have many uses. First, because of their high sugar content, they can be made into a sort of honey – a real treat for the sorely deprived sweet-toothed ancients. They can also be fermented to produce wine. If they are

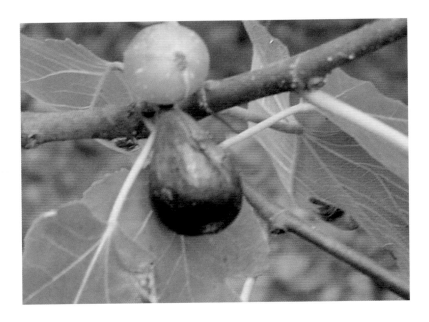

dried, they remain edible for a long time, which means that they are suitable for long journeys. Fig leaves can be smoked like tobacco. No part of the fig's fruit is wasted, and for this reason, it symbolizes the Torah: while all the other types of fruit contain inedible pits or peel, the fig, like the Torah, contains no bad parts.

It is said that the leaves of the fig were used to make the first clothes worn by Adam and Eve. Rabbi Nehemiah explains that the fig is also the Tree of Knowledge. Adam and Eve sinned by eating the fruit of the Tree of Knowledge, and they compounded their sin by using its leaves to make themselves clothes.

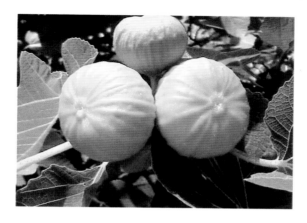

In folk medicine, eating dried figs is a sure remedy for constipation and many other digestive problems as well as anemia.

Boiling five figs in hot water, leaving them to soak in it for three days, then filtering the mixture results in a syrup that is effective in cases of poor digestion and anemia, as well as for curing coughs and colds. The recommended dosage is five spoonfuls a day.

The white milky liquid that seeps out of the fig's branches if they are broken is effective in treating welts and purulent wounds if applied several times. Five to ten drops of that same liquid can be mixed in hot water and applied to eye infections.

Funeral Cypress

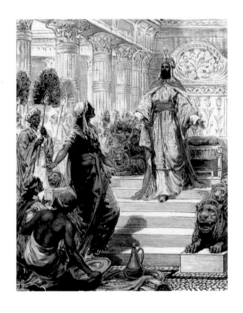

"Now King Hiram of Tyre having supplied Solomon with cedar and cypress timber and gold, as much as he desired, King Solomon gave to Hiram twenty cities in the land of Galilee."

I Kings 9:11

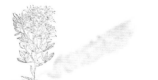

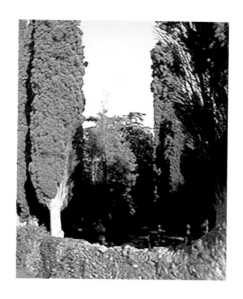

*T*he name of this proud evergreen tree, a symbol of height and firmness, does it a disservice. The cypress can reach a height of 100 feet, with a slender pointed top and dry, needle-like leaves. Before it was cultivated in order to form a buffer against harsh winds, it had a natural candle shape, and may have gotten its name from that, since it was often planted in cemeteries as a symbol of life. The cypress cones emerge in the spring.

It has numerous properties and uses. Its wood is strong, firm and enduring. Boats and ships were made of it in Tyre, and ancient houses whose roofs were made of cypress beams have been preserved until today, 15 centuries later. The walls of the Temple were made of cypress wood. This tree has an astonishing life-span of two millennia.

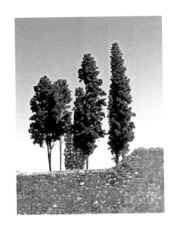

Visiting the Western Wall, one cannot miss the lovely cypresses that grow around it. These trees are almost as ancient as the Wall itself, and feature in many paintings of it throughout the ages. They are a symbol of strength and life and complement the Wall's majestic defiance of time.

Grind five cypress fruits to a powder and simmer it in water for about half an hour. Gargling with this mixture several times a day is an effective treatment for bleeding gums, toothache, caries, and loose teeth. About four spoonfuls of it help people who suffer from heartburn. Diabetics can benefit from drinking four glasses of water in which the cypress fruits have been boiled .

Cypress tea is highly effective in cases of digestive tract bleeding, normal or bloody diarrhea, and dysentery. All parts of the plant are a renowned folk remedy for stopping bleeding.

Garlic

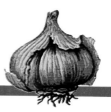

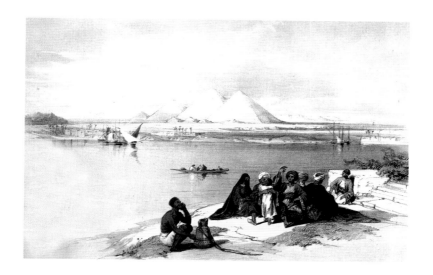

"We remember the fish, which we did eat in Egypt freely; the cucumbers, and the melons, and the leeks, and the onions, and the garlick."

Numbers 11:5

*F*amiliar to all aficionados of spicy food and horror fiction, the garlic plant has earned its place as a favorite modern herb and vampire repellant with its pungent aroma and numerous healing properties. Back in ancient Egypt, rumor has it that the slaves who built the pyramids fed mainly on garlic to maintain their strength. Some time later, Hippocrates mentioned it in his writings, and the Romans grew it in special gardens to feed the poor. The Chinese considered it a herb for cardiac ailments, and it is widely used today in food and medicine.

The garlic plant's narrow, grass-like leaves grow from its bulb, which is actually the edible part, and is ripe for picking in the fall. These leaves wrap around the single stem, which grows to a height of between one and three feet, ending in an umbel of pinkish flowers.

There are perhaps more superstitions and folklore linked to garlic than to any other plant. First there is the obvious vampire connection, as old as the myth itself: in the most desolate and isolated parts of Eastern Europe, villagers still hang clusters of garlic from their doorframes to keep the undead away. Garlic's power seems to extend to warding off all mystical misfortune; Homer relates that Odysseus used garlic to keep the witch Circe from turning him into a swine as she did to

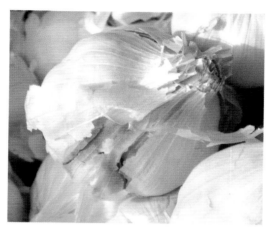

his crew. To the ancient Egyptians, garlic was an essential part of oath-taking. This may all seem strange in the light of one particular legend I know, in which garlic sprang up from the first step of Satan's left foot upon the earth when he left the Garden of Eden in Man's wake.

Garlic has a lengthy history as a medicinal herb, and science has verified many properties that have long been ascribed to it by popular belief. Eating three to six cloves of garlic a day fortifies the body and cleanses it. It is also helpful in preventing high cholesterol levels and high blood pressure, in healing respiratory and digestive diseases, and in easing many chronic conditions. It has proved to be a cure for colds and flu, for asthma and bronchitis, and for much more serious illnesses like dysentery and tuberculosis.

To make drops for ear infections, five cloves of garlic should be cooked in three spoonfuls of olive oil. Ground garlic can be applied to open wounds, infected gums and eyes, and aching teeth.

Grape

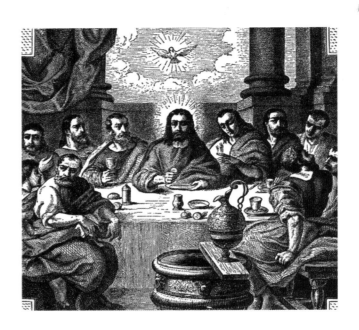

"I am the true vine, and my Father is the husbandman... Every branch in me that beareth not fruit he taketh away: and every branch that beareth fruit, he purgeth it, that it may bring forth more fruit."

John 15:1-2

"And they came unto the brook of Eshcol, and cut down from thence a branch with one cluster of grapes, and they bare it between two upon a staff; and they brought of the pomegranates, and of the figs."

Numbers 13:23

"Thou hast brought a vine out of Egypt: thou hast cast out the heathen, and planted it."

Psalms 80:8

"And Noah began to be an husbandman, and he planted a vineyard."

Genesis 9:20

T he grapevine, from which wine is produced to make men merry, is mentioned hundreds of times in the Scriptures. Along with the fig, its name comes up in every description of peace and prosperity. The abundance of the land, it seems, can be measured in its grapevines and the wine they produce. Even today, in many yards in Middle Eastern villages, the grapevine growing alongside a wall, shading a bench or shed, its crimson or green fruits hanging in great clusters and its scent in the air, evokes a peaceful and nostalgic atmosphere.

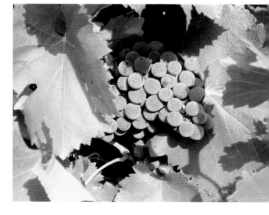

The wine that is produced from the grapes is a beverage that plays a great role in the history of mankind. Its pleasures were

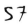

well known to the ancients, and its production and variety of types and customs have evolved into all but an art form. There are countless types of wine produced worldwide – some priced at tens of thousands of dollars for a single bottle. Wine was probably the first alcoholic beverage our ancestors learned to produce. Its production is actually very simple, and in the old days, when the grapes were crushed with the bare feet in a wild dance, it was an enjoyable process and a reason for celebration.

Wine was the main beverage of most Westerners until recent times – certainly more popular than water, which was very often polluted and not at all fit for drinking. I know at least two dozen versions of the story of the nobleman who demanded a drink, and, when he was given a glass of water, protested, outraged: "I wanted to drink, not to bathe!"

The grapevine has strong, stiff stalks and softer ones that grow and wrap around anything they can, pulling the plant upward and making it ideal as a natural roof or wall decoration. The leaves are large and rough to the touch, resembling a human hand in shape. In the spring, the vine blooms in clusters of tiny green flowers, which turn into the familiar juicy dark red or greenish fruits.

Naturalist medicine recommends fresh grape juice as a great source of vital minerals, such as calcium, iron, and potassium, as well as vitamins A, B1, B2 and C. Grapes speed up metabolism and digestion, making them more efficient and expediting the excretory process. The juice is also a good treatment for constipation and indigestion, anemia, skin diseases, and kidney problems.

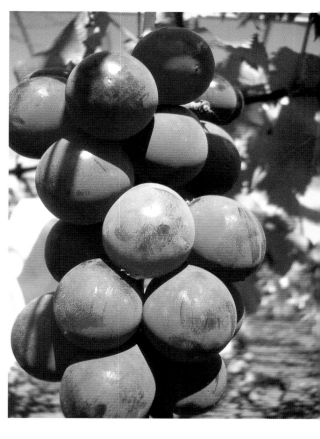

In Tunis, migraine sufferers wash their heads with grape vinegar. In Iraq, the leaves are burned and the ashes mixed with cold water to get rid of gallstones. In addition, the leaves are cooked in goat's milk and flax seeds to increase milk production in new mothers. In Morocco, wounds are bandaged with grape leaves, and among Yemenite Jews, drops of the liquid produced from cut grape's stalks are applied to eye infections.

Hairy Flax

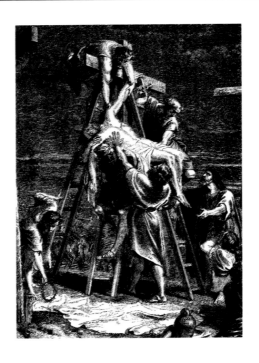

"They took they the body of Jesus, and wound it in linen clothes with the spices, as the manner of the Jews is to bury."

John 19:40

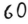

"And the flax and the barley was smitten: for the barley was in the ear, and the flax was bolled."

Exodus 9:31

"Thou shalt not wear a garment of divers sorts, as of woollen and linen together."

Deuteronomy 22:11

J n Biblical times, this plant was so important for the production of cloth and garments was so great that the word fabric was all but synonymous with its name. The hairy flax is a small bush, less than two feet high, with white stems covered in thin hairs. It blooms in great pink flowers in the spring.

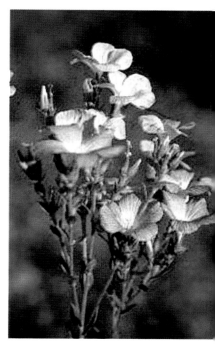

Producing fabric – linen – from the hairy flax is a lengthy operation. The stems must be dried, soaked in water, cracked and then combed until the thin fibers they contain have been removed. However, the hard work pays off – linen clothes are light and comfortable. They have been popular since the Stone Age some 10,000 years ago. Fishing nets and burial clothes were made of linen in ancient Egypt, and this tradition holds true today as well.

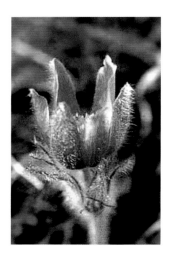

The priests of the Temple, who had to keep themselves perfectly clean, were permitted to wear only linen clothes so as to avoid sweating in the hot summers of the Holy Land. The body of Jesus, we are told, was buried in linen. Hairy flax and wool fulfilled all the ancients' textile needs. The plant was of such importance that in the Gezer Tablet, an ancient calendar, the 10th month is called "the month of picking flax".

In addition to the production of linen, the seeds of the hairy flax are edible. Oil with medicinal properties is produced from them. This oil was very precious in ancient times.

Another use of flax seeds is frying them and mixing them with honey. The resulting sweet mixture is effective in curing coughs, indigestion, and even impotence. Fried, ground and mixed with olive oil, the flax seeds make a thick ointment that can be applied to purulent wounds and pimples.

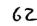

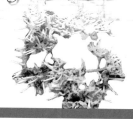

Henna

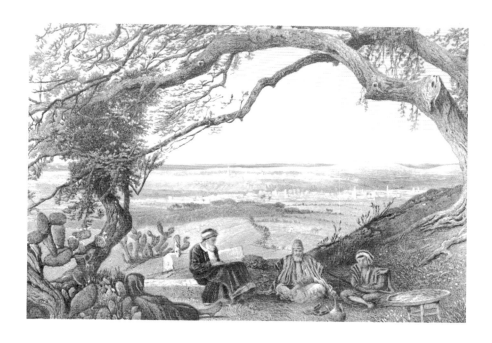

"My beloved is unto me as a cluster of camphire in the vineyards of En-gedi."

Song of Solomon 1:14

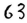

63

"Thy plants are an orchard of pomegranates, with pleasant fruits; camphire, with spikenard."

Song of Solomon 4:13

Originating from India, this bush or tree is best known for the red-brown dye that is produced from its ground leaves. Henna, or camphire, was used in ancient Egypt to paint the fingernails of mummified bodies, and later to dye fabrics and clothes. Further into Asia, henna is used to dye the hair and skin. Today, it is not uncommon to use henna for quick and easily removable tattoos, sometimes for ceremonial purposes. This is great for teenagers.

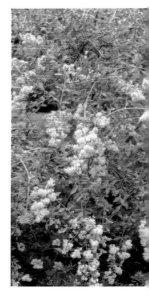

The henna plant, a thick, bushy tree, grows to a height of ten feet. It blooms in white, or sometimes red or yellow, and has simple leaves. Its flowers exude a heavy, seductive scent, especially in the evening. Its fruits, which contain many seeds, are ripe for picking all year round.

Jewish communities worldview employ the henna plant for various purposes. In Iraq, henna itself is applied in cases eczema, rashes, bleeding gums and measles. In Morocco, it is mixed with flour and egg yolk to

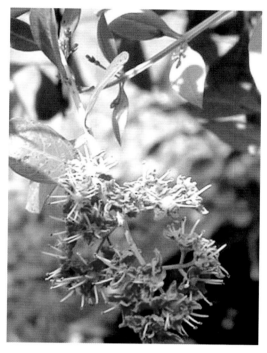

spread on broken limbs. Among the Jews of Tunisia, a teaspoonful of henna is boiled in water and drunk for seven days to regulate menstrual periods.

The following are folk remedies, and some are more reliable than others. One can mix green henna plant powder with ground pomegranate peel, add wine and spread the paste on burns, boils and open wounds. It also eases the pain of stiff joints. A teaspoonful of henna boiled in a cup of water can be used as a mouthwash for the treatment of bleeding gums and loose teeth.

Holy Bramble

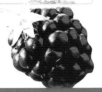

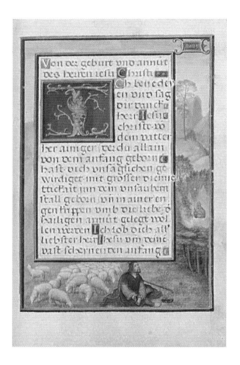

"And the angel of the Lord appeared unto him in a flame of fire out of the midst of a bush: and he looked and, behold, the bush burned with fire, and the bush was not consumed."

Exodus 3:2

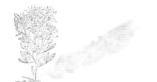
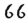

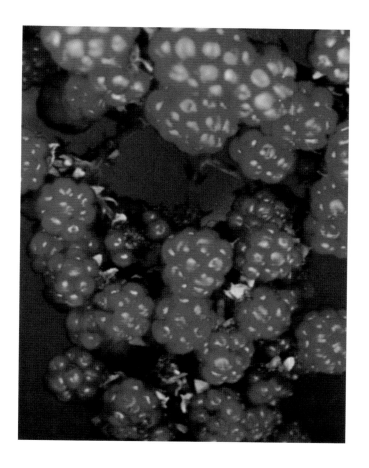

"And when the Lord saw that he turned aside to see, God called unto him out of the midst of the bush, and said, Moses, Moses. And he said, Here am I."

Exodus 3:4

*J*t is generally agreed that the holy bramble is in fact the famous burning bush by means of which God revealed himself to Moses in the desert. This thorny bush grows to a height of about seven feet with straight branches covered in hooked bumps that allow it to catch hold of nearby objects. Its small leaves are covered in smaller hooks, its flowers are a delicate pink, and it yields a fiery red berry-like fruit.

It is because of these fruits that some researchers think the holy bramble appeared to Moses to be burning. At sunset and sunrise, when red rays of light seem to endow it with a halo, it is a marvelous sight, and it is easy to believe that it is miraculously burning without being consumed. The holy bramble is not really a desert plant – it needs plenty of water to grow. For years, this mystery puzzled botanists, who could not understand how it could be the burning bush. The mystery was solved when it was discovered that Mt. Katarina and Mt. Sinai are much rainier areas than people thought – with snow as well.

The fruit of the holy bramble can be picked all year round and made into a sweet jam and a syrup with medicinal properties. To make the syrup, cook a pound of it in a pint of water. As it cooks, add 12 more ounces, and let the mixture cook over a low heat until it thickens. Two spoonfuls of this syrup will cure a cough and sore throat as well as diarrhea.

Another treatment for diarrhea, which is effective for ulcers as well, is cooking a handful of stems and leaves in a quart of water for half an hour.

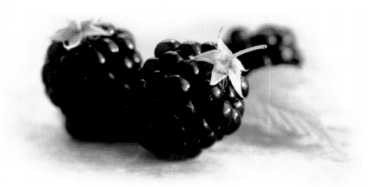

Filter the mixture, add honey to sweeten it, and drink two cups a day. The same mixture can be applied to inflamed gums: gargle with it six times a day.

Another option is a bramble bath. This involves cooking a pound grams of the holy bramble's branches and stems in two quarts of water for half an hour and adding the resulting filtrate to a bath of hot water. A half-hour soak is good for skin diseases, venereal infections, burns and hemorrhoids. Burns and chafing can also be cured with holy bramble leaves ground into a fine powder.

Hyssop

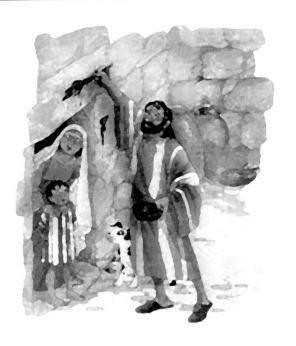

"And ye shall take a bunch of hyssop, and dip it in the blood that is in the bason, and strike the lintel and the two side posts with the blood that is in the bason; and none of you shall go out at the door of his house until the morning."

Exodus 12:22

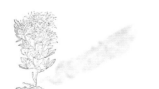

"And he shall cleanse the house with the blood of the bird, and with the running water, and with the living bird, and with the cedar wood, and with the hyssop, and with the scarlet."

Leviticus 14:52

"Now there was set a vessel full of vinegar: and they filled a spunge with vinegar, and put it upon hyssop, and put it to his mouth."

John 19:29

"And he spake of trees, from the cedar tree that is in Lebanon even unto the hyssop that springeth out of the wall: he spake also of beasts, and of fowl, and of creeping things, and of fishes."

I Kings 4:33

*H*yssop is a tiny plant whose small leaves contain many amazing qualities. It grows to a height of barely a foot, sends its roots snaking into rocks and limestone, climbs sheer rock walls, and hides humbly in their cracks. Its small gray-green leaves are soft to the touch, and exude a distinct spicy smell when crushed. It blooms in delicate white flowers in the heat of the summer, and conserves water by hiding from the sun among the rocks.

In Biblical times, hyssop was used in purification rites, possibly chosen for its pleasant smell as well as for its many true medicinal properties. Even

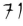

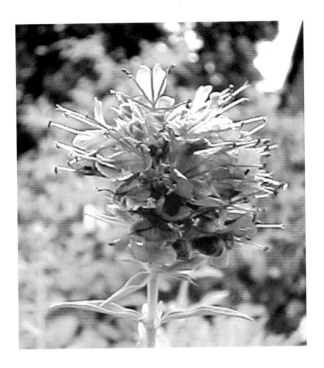

today, these rites are preserved among the Samaritans, where a priest dips the plant's thin branches into the blood of a sacrificial victim and sprinkles that blood on a person who has undergone purification. The Hebrews used branches of hyssop to smear the blood on their doorframes as a sign for the Lord to pass over their houses and spare their firstborn sons.

Rumor has it that among its many properties, the humble hyssop also keeps bad spirits as well as earthly pests of all sorts – ants and insects – at bay. Placing a bunch of hyssop on the table while eating is a lucky amulet.

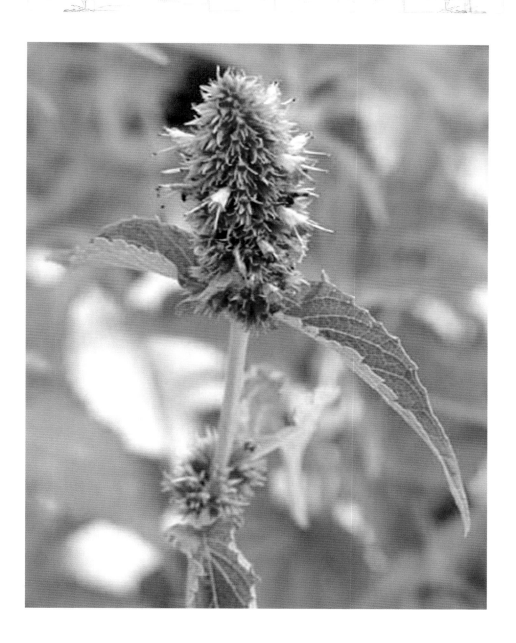

Hyssop is also quite good for eating – fresh, or as a delicious and widespread Middle Eastern herb.

Hyssop is one of the most important medicinal plants in many Jewish communities around the world, since it is used for treating a variety of maladies. To treat nausea and an upset stomach, a spoonful of fresh or dried leaves should be boiled in a cup of water and the mixture sweetened with honey. The mixture is then drunk.

Another treatment consists of half-filling a jar with olive oil and stuffing in hyssop leaves and branches until it is filled to the brim. The jar is then left in the sun for two weeks. The result is a medicinal oil that is good for stomach-aches as well as coughs, and can be applied to ear infections, too. Rubbing the oil into the temples alleviates headaches. It can also be spread between the fingers of people suffering from eczema and for treating cracked, peeling skin.

Hyssop can also be made into tea. Two teaspoonsful of dried leaves in a pint of boiling water are good for infections of the stomach, lungs and liver, and for fortifying the heart.

Juniper

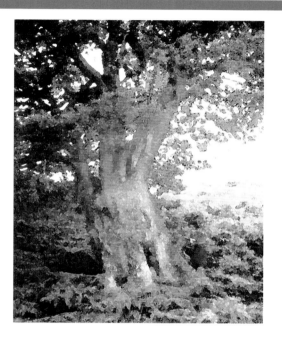

"*But he himself went a day's journey into the wilderness, and came and sat down under a juniper tree: and he requested for himself that he might die; and said, It is enough; now, o Lord, take away my life; for I am not better than my fathers.*"

I Kings 19:4

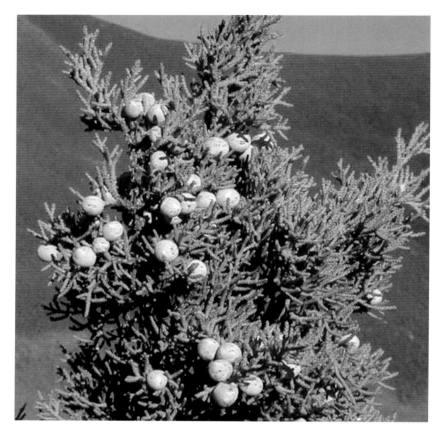

This is a pretty tree that grows to a height of between 20 and 40 feet and lives in the desert areas around the Jordan river. The juniper has straight branches stretching toward the sky and thick scaly leaves with jagged edges but blunt tips. They are dark or bluish green in color. Its fruits, which are glossy brown balls, can be picked all year round.

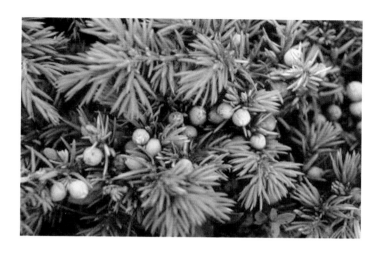

The juniper is used for making furniture and household items, since it is loved by carpenters everywhere for the delicate scent of its bark and roots. That same scent is used in the production of aromatic oils from the fruits and branches, oils that are also used to spice stiff drinks.

Almost 4,000 years ago, the juniper had medicinal uses in ancient Egypt, and it remains a folk remedy today. In the Jewish communities of South Africa, its black resin, which they call "Ketran", is used for treating recurring skin infections, and is a proven cure for eczema.

The juniper's round fruits are eaten to ease stomach-aches and soothe bloated stomachs. The oil from the fruit is used in the treatment of urinal tract infections, and can be massaged into aching muscles.

Madonna Lily

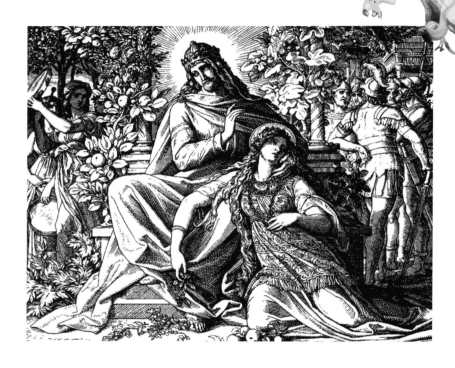

"I am a rose of Sharon, and the lily of the valleys. / As a lily among thorns, so is my love among the daughters."

Song of Solomon 2:1-2

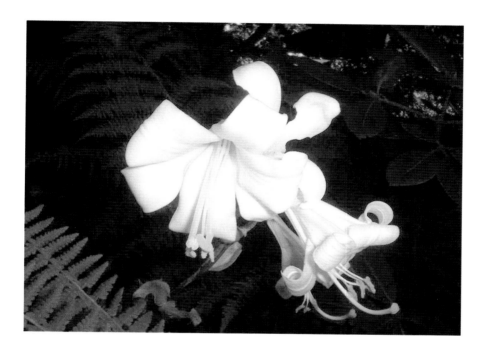

"My beloved is gone down into his garden, to the beds of spices, to feed in the gardens, and to gather lilies."

Song of Solomon 6:2

"Consider the lilies how they grow: they toil not, they spin not; and yet I say unto you, that Solomon in all his glory was not arrayed like one of these."

Luke 12:27

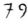

*T*his flower is one of the most commonly mentioned both in the Bible and the New Testament, appearing frequently in paintings of religious scenes. The beautiful Madonna lily reaches four feet in height and bears up to 20 great white flowers with gentle, curving petals that exude an intoxicating scent. During the winter, its leaves remain modestly hidden, spread on the ground, but in spring it blooms in all its tender glory.

Justifiably, Madonna lilies were considered to be the most beautiful of flowers. Their beauty was a metaphor for feminine beauty, as we see in the Song of Songs. Their shape inspired the shape of the Temple columns.

According to the legend, when Adam and Eve were banished from the Garden of Eden, Eve's bitter tears fell on the harsh ground, and from every tear rose a white lily. Among many ancient peoples, this delicate flower, which grows from among the thorns, was a symbol of all that is holy and pure.

The bulb of the lily is thought to be effective in treating injuries. Simmered in milk, it can be applied to skin infections, bruises and burns. A handful of flowers placed in a jar of olive oil and left in the sun for a month creates a liquid that can be massaged into the skin to ease headaches and backaches.

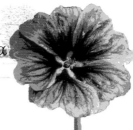

Mallow

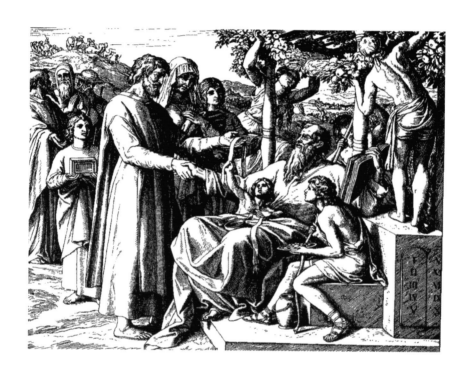

"Is there any flavor in the juice of mallows?"

Job 6:6

"Who cut up mallows by the bushes, and juniper roots for their meat."

Job 30:4

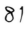

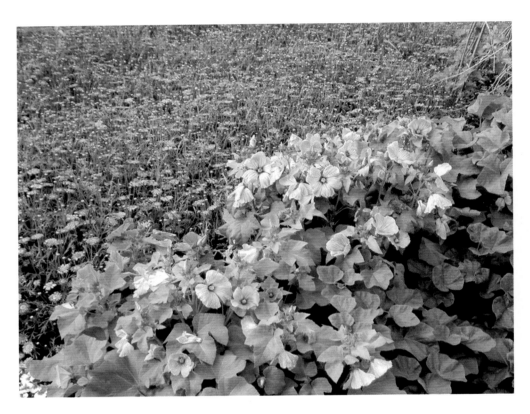

*T*he mallow is a low bush, about two feet high, and grows everywhere – at the side of the road, in small settlements, and in the wild. It is a hardy plant whose stalk is covered with thin hairs, and whose leaves are very large and soft with delicately jagged edges. Its flowers – pinkish blue lined in crimson – bloom from the top of the plant in the early spring. All year round, from January to June, it grows small round fruits that are divided into sections like a cake.

Not only is the mallow edible, but virtually every part of it, from the roots to the seeds, can be used to make a great variety of delicious foods. Arab shepherds and Israeli schoolchildren on class trips enjoy its fruits freshly picked. During Israel's War of Independence, when Jerusalem was under

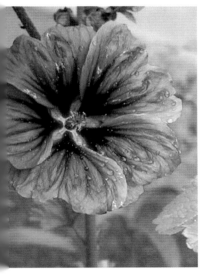

siege and running out of food supplies, the nutritious mallow plant became the city's mainstay and may well have saved it from being conquered.

The mallow plant contains a thick liquid with disinfectant properties and healing powers for respiratory, urinal, and vaginal diseases as well as necrosis. Simmer six ounces of leaves and in a pint of water for about 30 minutes. A viscous substance remains. Squeeze the water out into a glass, and process the remainder in a food processor with half a glass of olive oil.

Both the paste and the water are powerful remedies. The mallow paste can be applied to burns, necrotic and open wounds, and infected skin and rashes. The water is even more efficient as a cure for coughs and urinary tract and vaginal infections. Washing the hair with it strengthens the roots.

Finally, mallow leaves, eaten plain and green, are good for one's eyesight: it should be noted that mallow leaves contain twelve times more vitamin A than carrots.

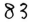

Mandrake

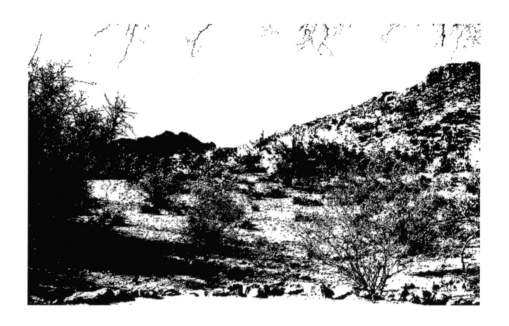

"And Reuben went in the days of wheat harvest, and found mandrakes in the field, and brought them unto his mother Leah. Then Rachel said to Leah, Give me, I pray thee, of thy son's mandrakes."

Genesis 30:14

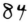

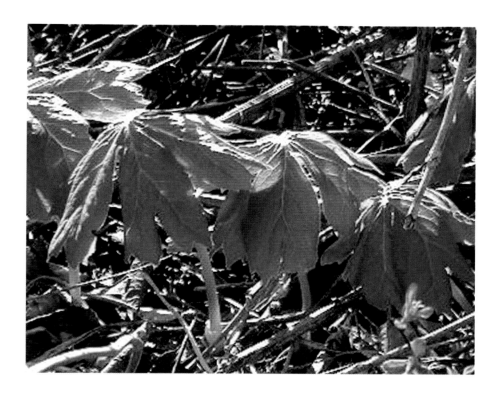

"The mandrakes give a smell, and at our gates are all manner of pleasant fruits, new and old, which I have laid up for thee, O my beloved."

Song of Solomon 7:13

*T*his small plant is a mixture of opposites: Above the ground, it is a small shrub less than a foot high. Below the ground, however, its root can be up to a yard long, and assume the surreal form of a human body. Its small, soft, purple flowers, blooming from the center of its cluster of wrinkled leaves, have an unpleasant smell, but this is not the case with its fruits. These golden-red balls have a lovely smell when they grow at the end of spring.

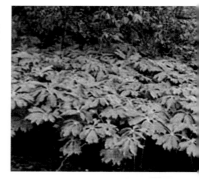

Despite their pleasant smell, the fruits do not have much of a taste. Moreover, they contain small amounts of poison, which, if consumed in substantial quantities, can cause madness. Hence the plant's Arabic name, the "madman's apple". That does not stop Arab shepherds from eating them during the harvest season.

According to legend, the mandrake can render barren men and women fertile. It may have been this legend that drove poor Rachel to all but trade her husband for the mandrakes in her desperation. This is a legend, however, which may stem from the spread "legs" of the anthropomorphic root. Nevertheless, when the mandrake's fruit is ground and mixed with garlic, it can be smeared on a bandage to ease the pain of a wound.

The Arabs of the Holy Land grind the root to a powder and apply it to snake bites. Two ounces of that powder, fried in olive oil, are rumored to be very helpful in such cases, as well as for the treatment of open wounds.

Myrtle

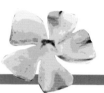

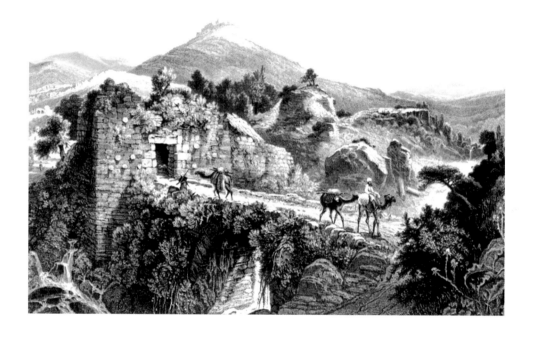

"...Go forth unto the mount, and fetch olive branches, and pine branches, and myrtle branches, and palm branches, and branches of thick trees, to make booths, as it is written."

Nehemiah 8:15

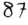

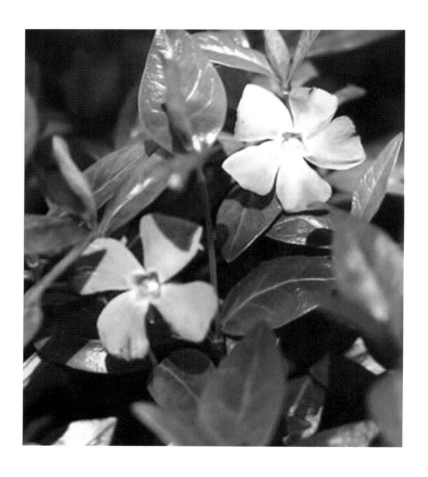

"*I will plant in the wilderness the cedar, the shittah tree, and the myrtle, and the oil tree; I will set in the desert the fir tree, and the pine, and the box tree together.*"

Isaiah 41:19

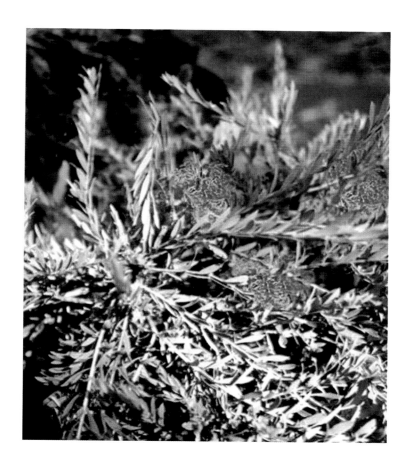

O ne of the sweetest-scented flowers known to man, the myrtle is a delicate plant about three feet high, with thin branches and soft, elongated, bright green leaves. Its marvelous flowers consist of a few white petals with a cluster of small stamens at their heart. The fruit is bluish black and reminiscent of a tiny pomegranate.

Thanks to its lovely scent, the myrtle has been one of the most important flowers in perfume-making from ancient times to this day. The Zohar [the Book of Splendor] calls its scent the most delicate of all scents on earth, capable of dispelling the foul stench of hell itself.

In Rome, the myrtle was a symbol of love, and brides wore it. Even today, the myrtle has a place of honor in many Jewish and Arab weddings.

The myrtle is one of the most important medicinal plants of the Holy Land and has numerous uses. Its leaves can be dried and ground to powder, which is mixed with olive oil to create a greenish ointment. This ointment relieves skin rashes, especially in babies, and, when massaged into the scalp, strengthens the roots of the hair to prevent it from falling out. When the ointment is placed on a bandage, it helps disinfect and heal bruises and open wounds. The powder can be put to similar use without the oil.

Fresh or dried myrtle leaves boiled in a cup of water make a pleasant tea, which can be sweetened with honey. This is an effective treatment for stomach infections, ulcers, and constipation. In Tunis and Algeria, this tea is also given to diabetics. Inhaling the steam of green myrtle leaves boiled in water helps asthma sufferers.

Oak

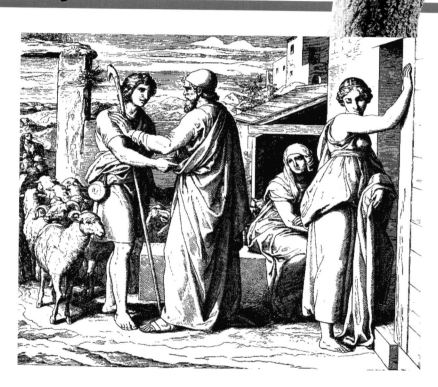

"And they gave unto Jacob all the strange gods which were in their hand, and all their earrings which were in their ears; and Jacob hid them under the oak which was by Shechem."

Genesis 35:4

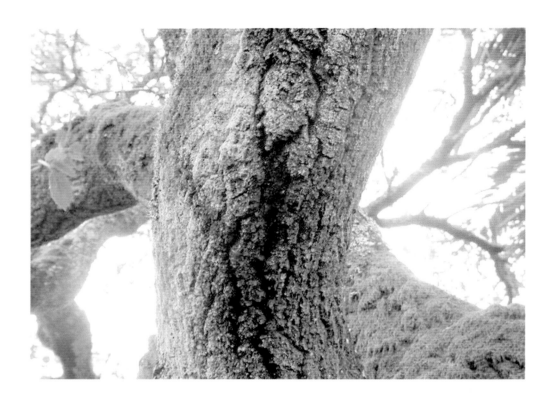

"And Absalom met the servants of David. And Absalom rode upon a mule, and the mule went under the thick boughs of a great oak, and his head caught hold of the oak, and he was taken up between the heaven and the earth; and the mule that was under him went away."

II Samuel 18:9

*T*he oak's Hebrew name stems from the root of the Hebrew word for "god", which goes to show how admired this tall, magnificent, tree was in ancient times. The oak tree grows to a great height, its trunk is very thick, and its rich, vast, green branches provide welcome shade. It produces greenish-yellow flowers in spring – March and April – on its smaller branches. In the autumn – between September and December – the familiar cone-shaped acorns in their thorny caps appear.

The oak used to cover most parts of the Holy Land, and is one of the trees most frequently mentioned in the Scriptures. It lives for many years. The Arabs consider it to be a symbol of eternal life, and the prophet Isaiah adopted it as one of his symbols of renewal. The roof of the Temple was made of huge oak beams, as were many pagan idols in ancient times.

Ten peeled acorns boiled in water for about half an hour result in a bitter liquid that helps prevent young children from wetting their beds. The dosage is half a glass before bedtime. For stomach-aches, simmer a teaspoonful of the flowers' yellow pollen in a quart of water and drink a glass of the liquid every day.

Four ounces of the oak's bark or its roots can be cooked in a quart of water for an hour to produce a strong tea that helps in cases of cancer of the digestive track. Two or three glasses a day are the recommended dosage.

Onion

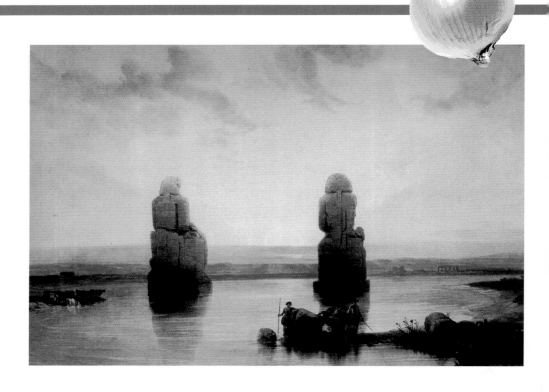

"We remember the fish, which we did eat in Egypt freely; the cucumbers, and the melons, and the leeks, and the onions, and the garlick."

Numbers 11:5

*T*he onion is one of the oldest cultivated plants known to man. Its name might come from the Latin word *unio*, meaning large pearl, because of its pearly white, multilayered bulb. Cylindrical, hollow leaves covered with a kind of wax, and – in the second year of the plant's life – the stem grow out of this bulb. The plant reaches a height of between two and four feet, devoid of leaves, its lower part hollow and swollen. At the top, the flowers are gathered in spherical clusters, greenish-white and with a strong green stripe traversing them.

Onions first became known in ancient Egypt as early as 3500 BCE, when they were grown and imported en masse to feed the slaves who were constructing the pyramids. Modern estimates for the price of these onions come to around three million dollars in ancient Egyptian currency. Almost 5,000 years ago, the Sumerians and Chinese grew them.

In many Mediterranean cultures, onions were an object of worship and an important part of pagan religion and symbolism. To the Egyptians, the onion's many peels and circle-within-a-circle structure were symbolic of eternal life, and there are actually paintings of onions on the inner walls of the great pyramids. Onions were used in the mummification process, and were buried alongside kings.

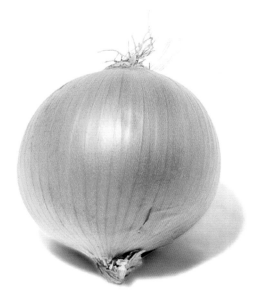

Placed on bandages and wrapped around the head, onions ease headaches. They also help wounds and bruises to heal. When ground, they alleviate the pain of bites and stings of all sorts. Mixed with salt, they make an effective painkiller. Onion juice mixed with olive oil can be applied to ear infections. Mixed with milk, it kills abdominal parasites. Plain juice onion cleanses and invigorates facial skin.

The healing power of the onion is evident in the lungs and digestive tract. It lowers blood pressure and promotes kidney function. Drinking its juice diluted with a lot of water has been known to help with allergies.

Peppermint

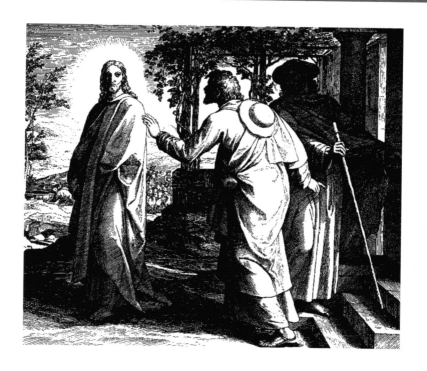

"But woe unto you, Pharisees! For ye tithe mint and rue and all manner of herbs, and pass over judgment and the love of God: these ought ye to have done, and not to leave the other undone."

Luke 11:42

97

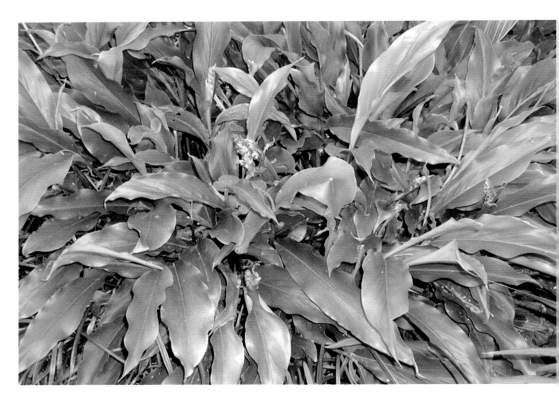

*A*lthough there are many types of mint, it is the peppermint that is most likely to be the one mentioned in the Scriptures. It is a small plant, between one and two feet high, with angular bluish stalks, and gently jagged, dark green leaves. The reddish, greenish and white flowers are small, and are arranged in a spearhead on the tops of the stalks. The peppermint is fairly common in gardens as a herb as well as for beauty.

Mint has a long history and a variety of uses. An ancient Greek myth links it to hospitality, telling of the elderly couple who used mint to spice a meal served to two travelers who turned out to be the gods Zeus and Hermes. The gods then rewarded the old man and woman by turning their home into a great temple.

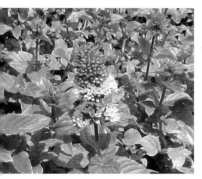

Another ancient use of the mint was for purposes of hygiene. Mint was used to make bathwater and soap fragrant. In the 14th century, people used mint to whiten their teeth; today its distilled oil is still used to flavor toothpaste.

In the Mediterranean, peppermint is used in folk medicine as a treatment for many ailments from eye infections to impotence. A handful of peppermint leaves boiled in water for ten minutes makes a spicy, marvelously healthy tea, which is very effective against chronic tiredness, headaches, stomach-aches, nausea, and vomiting. It can also be applied to eye infections and swellings, and can lower fever in small children. Mixed with a little wine, it prevents halitosis and oral infections.

Tea made of the peppermint's stalks cures many digestive diseases. Finally, a handful of crushed leaves can be put in a bottle full of sunflower oil, and the bottle left on a sunny windowsill for ten days. It should be shaken occasionally, and strained thoroughly at the end of the duration. The oil can be massaged into the temples to ease powerful migraines.

Pistachio

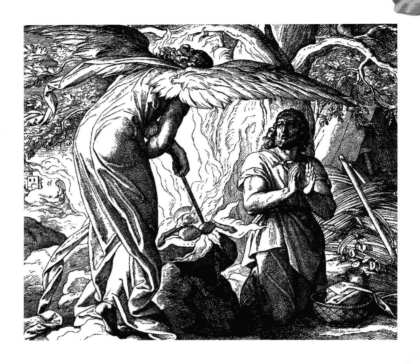

"And there came an angel of the Lord, and sat under an oak which was in Ophrah, that pertained unto Joash the Abi-ezrite: and his son Gideon threshed wheat by the winepress..."

Judges 6:11

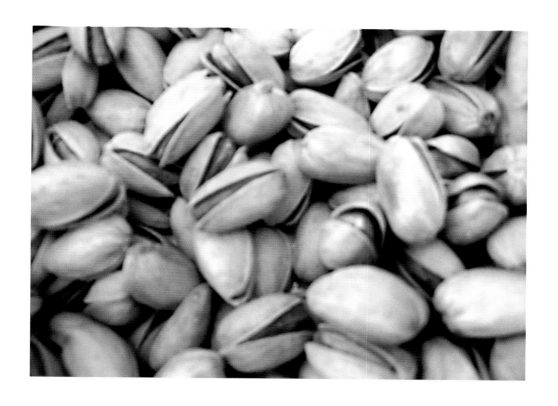

"For ye shall be as an oak whose leaf fadeth, and as a garden that hath no water."

Isaiah 1:30

As with the oak, this tree was linked to manifestations of deities, and worshiped as a deity itself in ancient times. Their names are often interchanged in translation. This bush can grow into a 20-foot-high tree with a thick trunk and a wide, proud top. Its elongated leaves first grow in the spring, sporting a reddish shade that returns before they fall off in the fall. The fruits change color from red to purple as they ripen in summer.

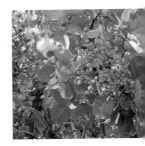

The pistachio was considered a sacred tree; the ancient Hebrews learned to worship it from the pagan peoples of Canaan, and its sanctity survived long into monotheism. Under its leaves, the Lord's messenger came to Gideon, and the judges of Israel sat in its shade during Mishnaic times. Today, the pistachio is appreciated less for its spiritual value than for the simple delight of its fruits.

The gummy resin of the pistachio is sold in spice markets. The ancients used it to combat halitosis, but chewing it and swallowing its juice is also a good remedy for stomach-aches, indigestion, ulcers, and heartburn. The same is true for the leaves, which also alleviate toothaches.

Two teaspoonfuls of pistachio bark boiled in water for half an hour have been known to halt internal bleeding, especially in the uterus. Soaking the hands or feet in the mixture is good for the treatment of eczema.

Pomegranate

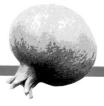

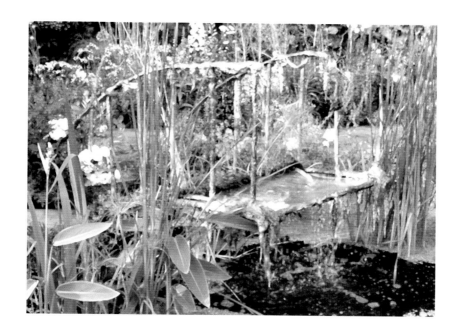

"I went down into the garden of nuts to see the fruits of the valley, and to see whether the vine flourished, and the pomegranates budded."

Song of Solomon 6:11

103

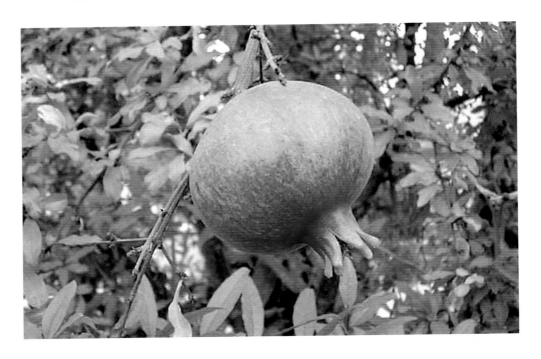

"The vine is dried up, and the fig tree languisheth; the pomegranate tree, the palm tree also, and the apple tree, even all the trees of the field, are withered: because joy is withered away from the sons of men."

Joel 1:12

"And wherefore have ye made us to come up out of Egypt, to bring us in unto this evil place? it is no place of seed, or of figs, or of vines, or of pomegranates; neither is there any water to drink."

Numbers 20:5

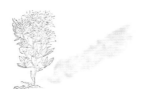

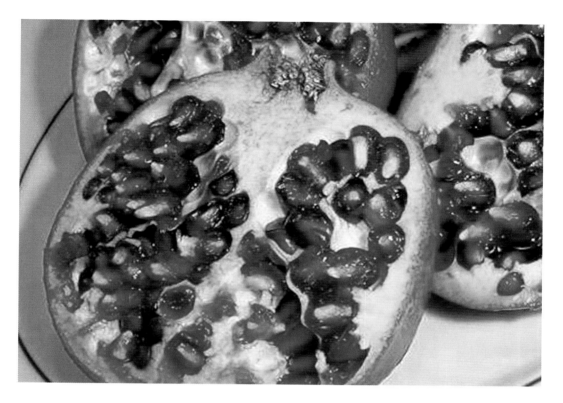

The pomegranate is a sweet fruit that originated in Persia and spread throughout the Middle East. Familiar to the ancient Hebrews, it was mentioned as one of the many blessings of the Holy Land. The pomegranate is a domesticated plant grown in orchards all around Israel. The tree grows to a height of between 10 and 20 feet, with numerous branches and a reddish tinge to its leaves. In the spring, it blooms in fiery red bells, and five weeks later, the round, glossy fruits are ripe, still bearing the crown shape of the flowers.

The pomegranate fruit consists of white pulp containing countless small red grains that house the seeds. They are so numerous that they have become a metaphor. Seated around the table during Rosh Hashana, the Jewish New Year, the family prays that "our good deeds be as numerous as the grains of the pomegranate". However, the pomegranate is not only linked to good deeds… its red bloom and fruits also symbolize lust and passion.

The peel of the pomegranate can be ground to powder and applied to minor injuries and boils, especially in babies and young children. That same powder can also be boiled in water – a teaspoonful per cup – and drunk in order to treat diarrhea, dysentery and other digestive problems. For inflamed gums and oral infections, three spoonfuls of powder should be boiled in two cups of water and the resulting mixture used for gargling.

Another traditional use of the pomegranate is mixing its juice with mint tea as a remedy for vomiting. Its ground peel can also be mixed with henna to produce a dark hair dye.

Rue

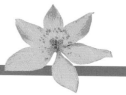

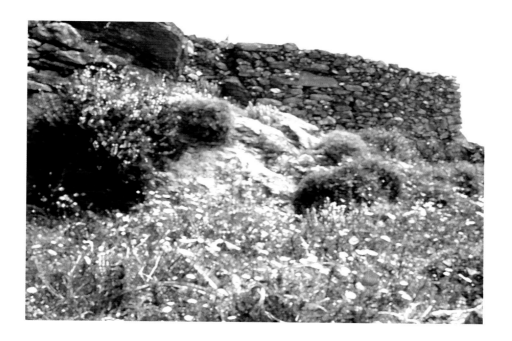

"But woe unto you, Pharisees! For ye tithe mint and rue and all manner of herbs, and pass over judgment and the love of God: these ought ye to have done, and not to leave the other undone."

Luke 11:42

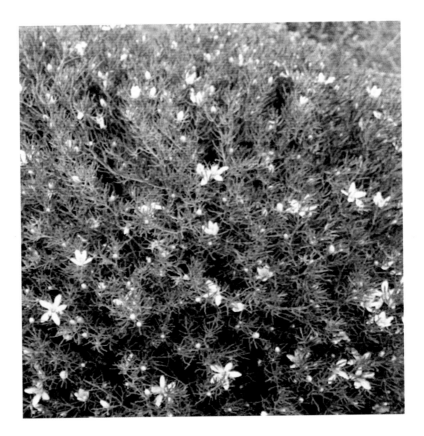

A nother ancient medicinal herb, rue was well known to the ancient Greeks, who gave it its name from a root meaning "to set free" because of its effectiveness in treating many diseases. Later, the Romans spread it on the floor of public buildings and walked around the streets carrying bunches of it for protection against illness.

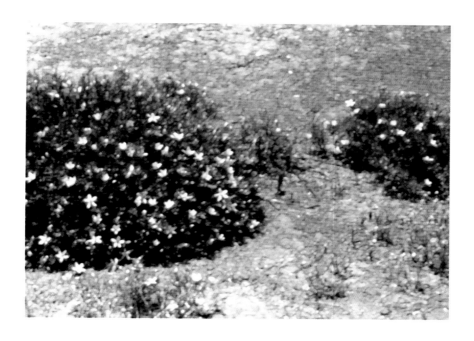

In medieval Europe, rue was the "plant of grace", a symbol of God's grace for the faithful who have repented for their sins. Its branches were once used for sprinkling holy water at the ceremony preceding High Mass, and it was thought to ward off the ill effects of witchcraft and black magic. It was considered a surefire way to be rid of fleas and pests. In addition, anyone who carried a branch of rue would be spared from contracting plagues. In courts, judges would put rue on the court bench to avoid contracting infections from sick prisoners.

109

In the Mediterranean, branches of rue are placed in front of a couple at their wedding, and in a baby's cradle to keep harm away. Because of its powerful scent and the shape of its leaves, it is still considered a talisman of good luck and a safeguard against demons and evil spirits.

Rue is a bush about three feet high with widespread, softly curving branches and delicate leaves shaped like a human hand. Its bright yellow flowers are arrayed in umbel-like clusters, and its fruit is a round pod full of seeds. The upper parts of the plant produce an aromatic oil that is responsible for the rue's powerful scent, which chases bugs and other animals – especially cats – away, making it very effective as an insect repellant.

Rue oil is a highly efficient cure for backaches, aching joints, and rheumatism when it is massaged into the aching limb, as well as headaches when it is rubbed on to the temples. It also cures ear infections, and is rumored to ease coughs in children when it is rubbed into their chests. It is produced by filling a bottle half with olive oil and half with leaves and stalks of rue, placing the bottle in a pot of water, and bringing the water to the boil. The oil is best applied warm.

Leaves and stalks of rue can also be boiled in water to produce a cure for stomach infections and indigestion. It is also effective for treating infections when it is rubbed gently over the eyelid. Washing the hair with it gets rid of lice.

Saffron

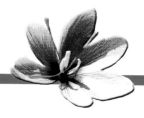

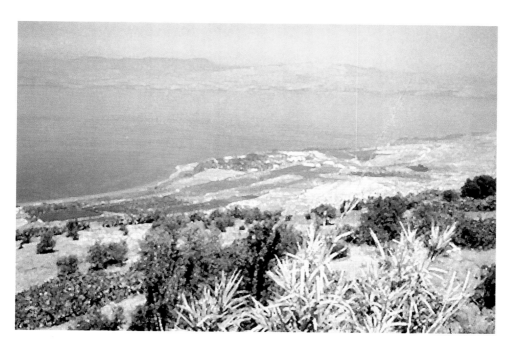

"Spikenard and saffron; calamus and cinnamon, with all trees of frankincense; myrrh and aloes, with all the chief spices."

Song of Solomon 4:14

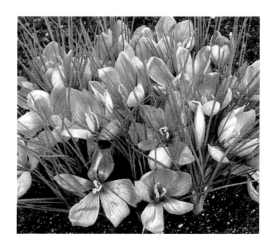

*T*his flower possesses two kinds of beauty: internal and external. Its external beauty lies in its large flowers, while its internal beauty resides in the expensive yellow dye that is produced from it. Saffron is a small plant with narrow, straight leaves that grow in a rosette. While its seeds are infertile, its bulblets spread around it. A single beautiful blue or white flower blooms from among the leaves. However, only the blue flowers produce the saffron dye.

Since ancient times, more than four millennia ago, the saffron has been grown as a spice, a dye and a garden flower. It takes about 4,000 saffron flowers to produce an ounce of the dye, which explains its astronomical price. It was used to spice wine in Biblical times and to perfume the air at weddings and in ancient Greek amphitheaters. The Assyrians used it to banish the evil spirits that haunt women in childbirth, and during the Middle Ages, many a scholar praised saffron for its effectiveness in love potions.

Nowadays, saffron has a less illustrious but equally useful role: it adds color to many foods, most notably oriental dishes such as curry. I remember a children's story about a king who decided he would eat nothing that was not yellow, and his desperate cook was rescued by a saffron flower that offered him its pollen to spread on the food. When the king came out of his palace to thank the flower, he saw the flowers of the field and his eyes were opened once more to the beauty of all the colors.

About a fifth of a teaspoonful of saffron fibers boiled in a glass of water for ten minutes produce a pain-relieving remedy for swellings, bruises, and wounds if a bandage is soaked in the mixture and applied. The mixture is also effective in the case of eye infections.

The fibers can also be boiled into a sort of tea – twenty fibers per cup of water. It is a good idea to add honey for taste and to drink the mixture as a treatment for liver diseases, colds, constipation, regulating menstrual periods, and in anticipation of giving birth. Gargling with the mixture counters halitosis.

Quite a few other folk medicines are made of saffron. Saffron tea is supposed to lower fevers, help in cases of impotence, and calm the body and mind before going to sleep. In India, the flowers are cooked in hot milk that is then drunk or spread around the nostrils to ease colds. A mixture of saffron and citron is said to fortify the heart.

Spotted Golden Thistle

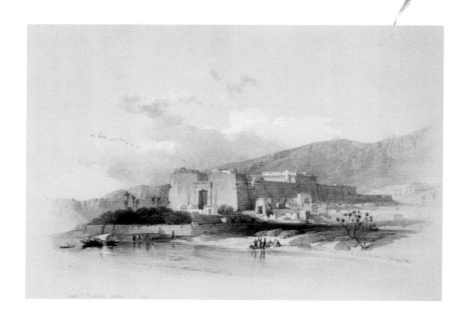

"As the lily among the thorns, so is my love among the daughters."
Song of Solomon 2:2

114

J f the Madonna lily is a symbol of all that is pure, the thistle is a symbol of perdition, desolation, and torment. Wherever it appears in the Scriptures, it is inevitably linked to some great punishment. The ground issues thistles to punish Adam and Eve. The growth of thistles in the field always symbolizes the ultimate fall and despair.

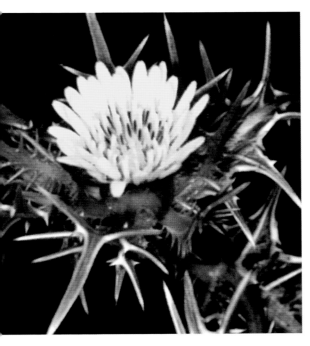

However, the golden thistle, one variant of many thorny plants, is also a medicinal herb. Its bright golden flowers grow on four-foot-high stems that are covered with thorny, white-rimmed leaves. Israeli Arabs boil the stems in water to make an important folk remedy. The stems should be peeled to prevent a bitter taste, cut into slices and cooked for 15 minutes. Four glasses a day work wonders for stomach-aches.

An ointment can be made from the golden thistle's seeds, fried lightly, ground and mixed with olive oil. The thick paste can be applied to open wounds or rubbed into the scalp if there are small wounds there. It can be stored in a sealed jar, and remains effective for a long time.

Tamarisk

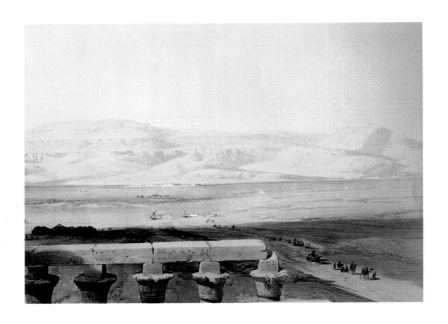

"And they took their bones, and burned them under a tree at Jabesh, and fasted seven days."

I Samuel 31:13

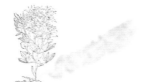

116

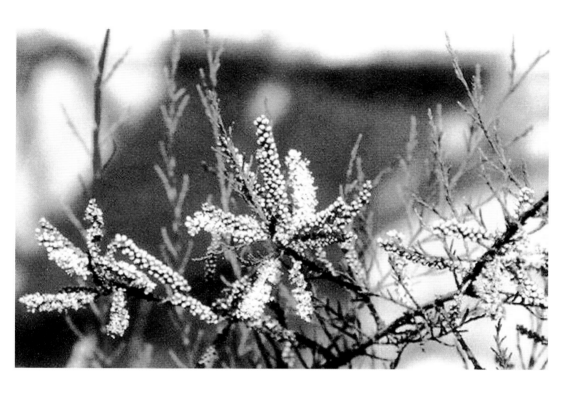

"And Abraham planted a grove in Beer-sheba, and called there on the name of the Lord, the everlasting God."

Genesis 21:33

J n the Holy Land, there are several species of tamarisk that play a part in a number of Biblical stories. They are so named in the Hebrew original. The healing qualities are those of the giant tamarisk. This tall tree grows all over the south of the country, reaching a height of 40 feet at times. Its trunk is wide and grayish, and its tiny leaves grow thickly and hug the branches to avoid losing water in the hot climate of the Negev. Its small white flowers bloom in the fall, between August and November.

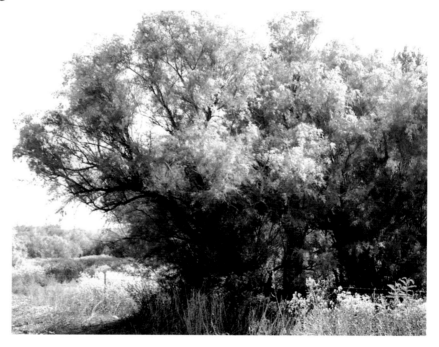

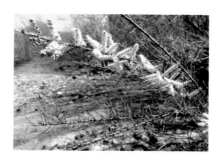

The tall, desert-dwelling tamarisk is planted as a monument – Abraham planted one in Beer Sheba, and the bones of Saul and his sons were buried in its sparse shade. Scientists today also link the tamarisk with the manna that the Hebrews ate in the desert. Tiny aphids feed on the tamarisk's flesh, leaving clean sugar on the bark in their wake and providing abundant food in the desert.

An infusion made from the tamarisk's leaves is renowned for its effects on pregnant women in folk medicine. Drinking it helps ease post-partum cramps, expedites the expulsion of the afterbirth, and cleanses the uterus. Four or five glasses a day of the infusion helps people who suffer from ulcers.

For a rinse against lice, eight ounces each of the tamarisk's bark and roots can be cooked together for a half-hour. A pint of vinegar should be added three minutes before the end of the cooking, and the hair should be rinsed with the resulting mixture after washing. This is a completely natural and effective replacement for a chemical treatment against lice.

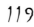

Thorny Caper

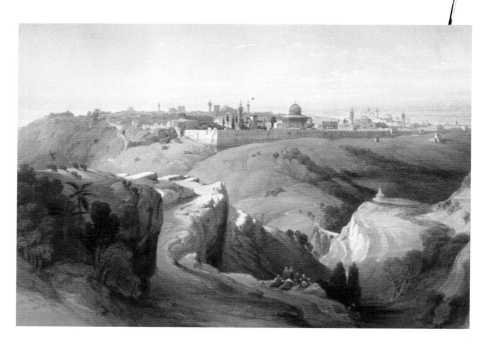

"Also when they shall be afraid of that which is high, and fears shall be in the way, and the almond tree shall flourish, and the grasshopper shall be a burden, and desire shall fail: because men goeth to his long home, and the mourners go about the streets."

Ecclesiastes 12:5

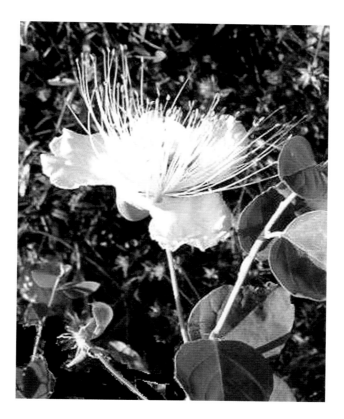

M entioned only once in the Scriptures – as "desire" – the thorny caper is a unique plant. Its favorite home is sheer walls or piles of rocks, snaking out from among old stones, seemingly needing no soil to sink its roots into. It can grow to a height of between two and six feet, stretching itself over the stone. Its arched stems bear roughly round, fleshy leaves, at whose base grows a pair of vicious, hooked thorns.

Its flowers are an amazing sight: they are large and consist of two flat white petals that enclose a cluster of pink stamens. It is strange and beautiful, and blooms between March and August. The buds are edible, as are the fruit and even the young branches. The caper was grown exactly for this purpose in the Talmud period.

The legend of how capers came into being tells of a boy – a gifted archer – who would not retreat behind the walls when the Greeks came to conquer Jerusalem. Boldly he stood and fought until he was shot down. His body then became a thorny plant that cannot be separated from the wall it is guarding.

The caper has been used since ancient times and is still used among Israeli Arabs to treat hearing problems, open wounds, toothaches, and even diabetes. The caper root is cooked in olive oil, and the oil is then applied to ear infections or to ears that are hard of hearing. This remedy works wonders on elderly people whose hearing is deteriorating.

The paste made of a ground caper leaf can be applied to ease toothaches. When boiled in a tea, the leaf helps diabetics. A bath can be filled with water in which caper leaves and stalks have been boiled – a half-hour's soak eases open and infected wounds and respiratory diseases, and is rumored to be effective in cases of female infertility.

Tumble Thistle

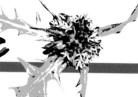

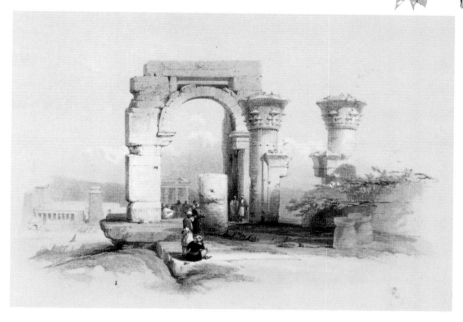

"O my God, make them like a wheel; as the stubble before the wind."

Psalms 83:13

"The nations shall rush like the rushing of many waters: but God shall rebuke them, and they shall flee far off, and shall be chased as the chaff of the mountains before the wind, and like a rolling thing before the whirlwind."

Isaiah 17:13

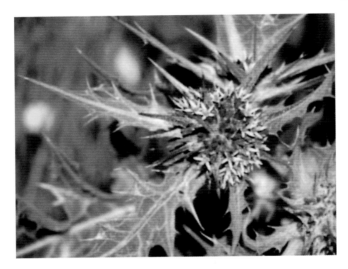

oubtlessly seeming to be one of the least pleasant plants in the Scriptures, the tumble thistle's thorny appearance is deceptive. It is a small bush, barely more than a foot high and not much wider, with thick stems spread on the ground. Its leaves are tough and spiky, so that access to its seeds is both difficult and painful. The seeds, which ripen between December and June, are large and edible – even tasty – and contain a lot of oil.

The name of the plant derives from the fact that during late fall, when its seeds are ripe, the plant becomes detached from its roots and dries up. Any powerful gust of wind then tears it up and sends it tumbling along. In a storm, the frenzied flight of the thistle is something to see, so much so that the Bible made it into a metaphor for uncontrolled flight and speed. There is a myth of a man who killed his cousin during a journey; there were no witnesses but the tumble thistle, which blooms in the spring. However, when the murderer returned to his village in the fall, the tumble thistle was carried there on the wind with him, and told all the villagers of his evil deed.

Arab farmers consider the tumble thistle a delicacy. With the first rains, they pick it and cook its thick root in a stew with meat and onions. The leaves can also be eaten; they are a good addition to a salad – so long at the plant is young and not too thorny! Simply eating the plant when it is young and green is enough to fortify the digestive system and ward off and cure diseases.

To treat liver diseases, simmer four ounces grams of the thistle's leaves and stalks in a quart of water for 15 minutes. Drink three glasses of the filtrate a day.

The tumble thistle's seeds can also be made into a tea that helps alleviate nausea, dizzy spells, allergies, and low blood pressure. Three spoonfuls of seeds should be boiled in a quart of water, and the dosage is five spoonfuls a day.

Twisted Acacia

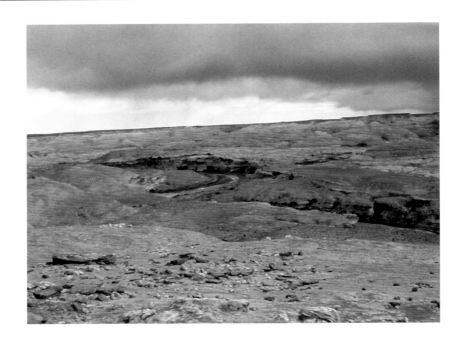

"I will plant in the wilderness the cedar, the shittah tree, and the myrtle, and the oil tree; I will set in the desert the fir tree, and the pine, and the box tree together."

Isaiah 41:19

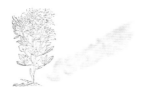

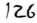

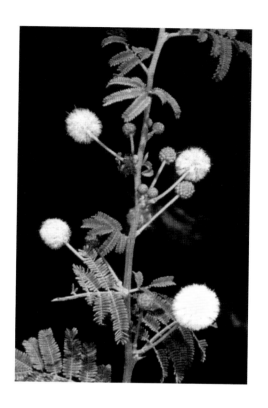

"And rams' skins dyed red, and badgers' skins, and shittim wood,"

Exodus 25:5

"And I made an ark of shittim wood and hewed two tables of stone like unto the first, and went up into the mount, having the two tables in mine hand."

Deuteronomy 10:3

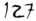

127

"And he made boards for the tabernacle of shittim wood, standing up."

Exodus 36:20

Growing in the desert, the acacia, the Biblical shittah, has a rough trunk that divides into several thick branches that can reach a height of 15 feet. Its leaves feature two small thorns growing at their base. The acacia blooms in October, with the first rains, producing small, round, bright yellow flowers.

The acacia is renowned for its use in the construction of the Tabernacle and its accessories. All of the wooden components were made from acacia wood, since it is the only tree that grows in relative abundance in the desert. Later, however, a tree that was used for a holy purpose out of necessity became a symbol of renewal in the visions of Isaiah.

The medically useful part of the acacia is its resin. Two teaspoonfuls of resin cooked in a quart of milk and drunk three times a day, between meals, is good for coughs, pulmonary bleeding, stomachaches, internal infections, and kidney stones.

The liquid resin can be mixed with an egg yolk and applied to open, bleeding wounds. In its semi-solid, gummy form, a lump of resin can be chewed to strengthen weak teeth.

walnut

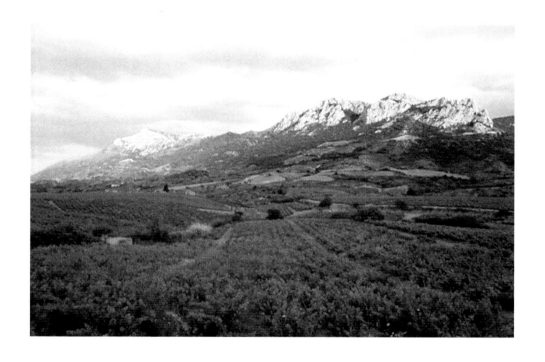

"I went down into the garden of nuts to see the fruits of the valley, and to see whether the vine flourished, and the pomegranates budded."

Song of Solomon 6:11

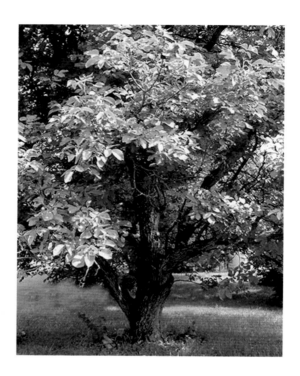

A tall, regal tree first cultivated in the Near East, the walnut tree stands over 40 feet high with a broad umbrella of branches. It is one of the last trees to bloom – in late spring – its leaves and green-yellow flowers appearing at the same time. Its round, wrinkled fruit, from which good oil is produced, ripens in the winter.

In the Hebrew, Greek, and Roman traditions, the walnut symbolizes the unity of a married couple. Throwing and scattering the nuts and their shells in front of the bride and groom at a wedding is a blessing of fertility and good fortune.

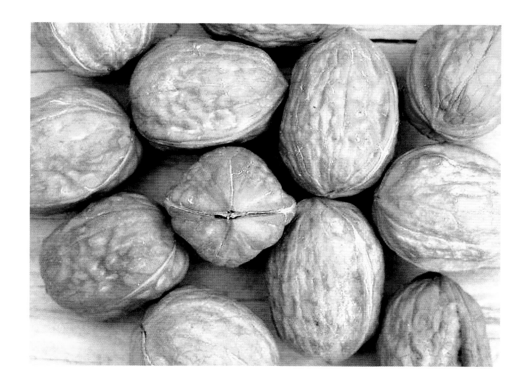

Naturalist medicine tells us that while the nut is still green, its peel can be squeezed to extract a clear liquid that is good for treating eczema and skin infections. Five drops of that liquid in half a cup of water are effective in the treatment of eye infections. A compress containing the liquid should be placed it on the eye. Scrubbing the teeth with the bark of the tree cleans them and makes them very white.

131

Watermelon

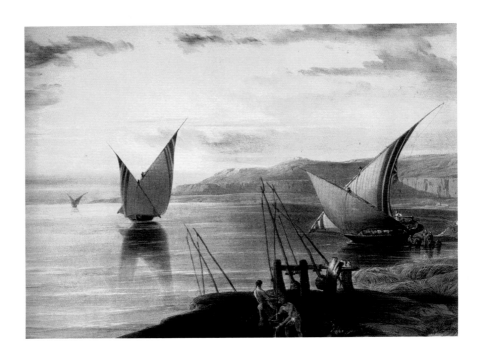

"We remember the fish, which we did eat in Egypt freely; the cucumbers, and the melons, and the leeks, and the onions, and the garlick."

Numbers 11:5

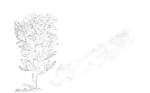
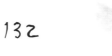

132

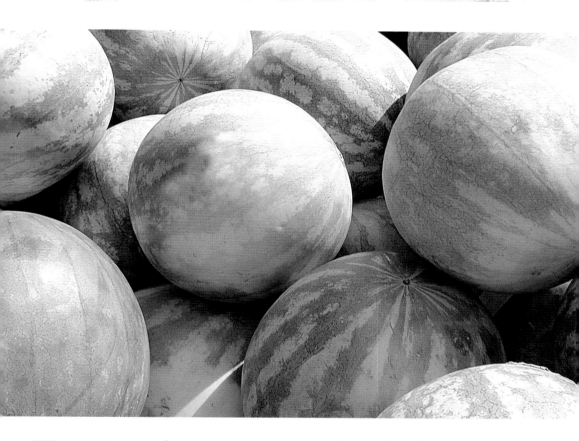

*I*t may be strange to encounter a fruit as familiar and banal as the watermelon in the Scriptures, yet it was evidently a popular summer treat for the ancient Egyptians. Paintings of watermelons were found from the time of the 21st dynasty of Egypt, over 3,000 years ago. It seems to have been an inexpensive, widely available fruit. Small wonder that its juicy memory haunted the Hebrews in the desert.

The watermelon plant grows outward on the ground, its elongated branches and the lower part of its green-gray leaves covered in thin hairs. Yellow flowers grow from within the leaves from May to August, and, between June and August, turn into the immense round fruit.

The watermelon has a marvelous affect on the bladder – three glasses of its juice a day, squeezed from the peel as well as the pulp, are good for any problem in that organ. Its juice also promotes liver function. Naturalist healers claim that the rich juice cleanses the kidneys and stimulates the appetite.

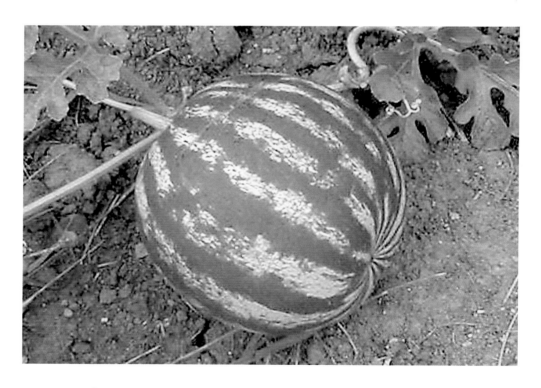

wheat

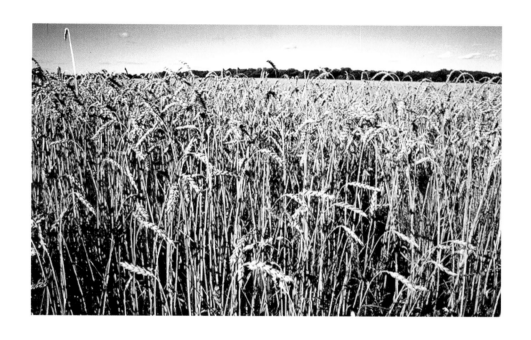

"Very truly, I tell you, unless a grain of wheat falls into the earth and dies, it remains just a single grain; but if it dies, it bears much fruit."

John 12:24

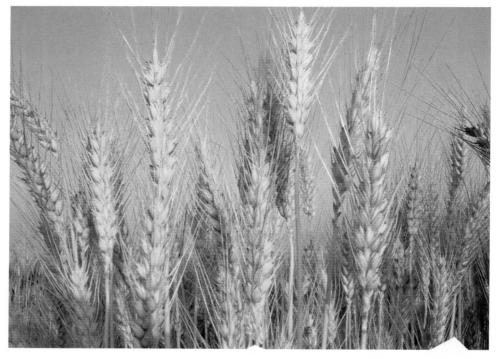

"He should have fed them also with the finest of the wheat: and with honey out of the rock should I have satisfied thee."

Psalms 81:16

"And Solomon gave Hiram twenty thousand measures of wheat for food to his household, and twenty measures of pure oil: thus gave Solomon to Hiram year by year."

I Kings 5:11

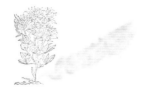
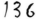

136

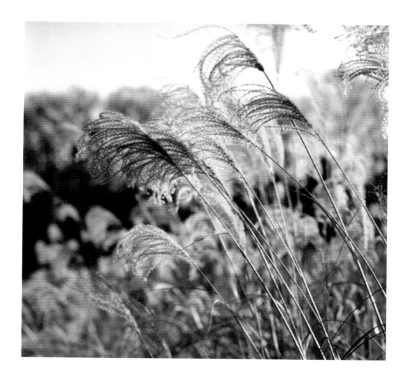

*P*ossibly the most important plant known to man, wheat is where bread comes from, Mother Earth's bounty. The image of golden fields of ripe wheat is the very essence of nostalgia, peace, and prosperity. Countless myths and metaphors surround its growth, its reaping, the harvest season, and breadmaking. Although wheat is most commonly ground to make flour, it may also be eaten freshly picked, nature's gift to laboring man.

137

Wheat grows in tall, straight stalks, its flowers in ears on their tips, ripening from green at the beginning of spring – March and April – to gold at the height of the harvest season from June to August. It is then peeled, dried and ground into flour.

Among its many merits, wheat fortifies the body, enriches the blood, improves digestion, and is good for the kidneys and bladder and for curing rashes and coughs. Water in which wheat grains have been cooked for an hour eases coughs and serves as a diuretic.

Even more useful, however, is the wheat's bran. Cook four ounces grams of it in water for an hour, add a cup of concentrated vinegar or the juice of unripe grapes, and drink one cup a day. This is a good remedy for increasing strength and vigor, for to enhancing milk production in women, and for dissolving kidney stones. Skin infections and allergic rashes can be treated by washing and massaging the infected limb with the mixture.

Wormwood

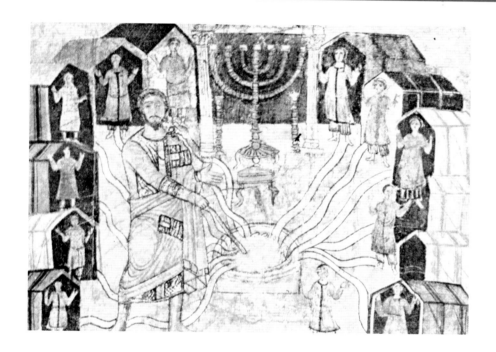

"Lest there should be among you man, or woman, or family, or tribe, whose heart turneth away this day from the Lord our God, to go and serve the gods of these nations; lest there should be among you a root that beareth gall and wormwood."

Deuteronomy 29:18

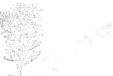

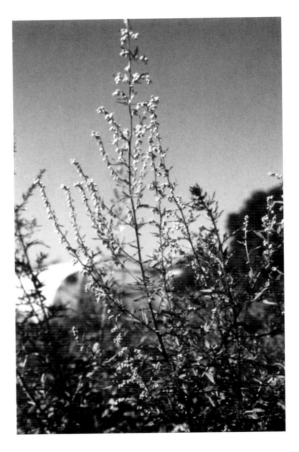

"Therefore thus saith the Lord of hosts, the God of Israel; Behold, I will feed them, even this people, with wormwood, and give them water of gall to drink."

Jeremiah 9:15

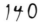

"Therefore thus saith the Lord of hosts concerning the prophet; Behold, I will feed them with wormwood, and make them drink the water of gall: for from the prophets of Jerusalem is profaneness gone forth into all the land."

Jeremiah 23:15

"Ye who turn judgment to wormwood, and leave off righteousness in the earth,"

Amos 5:7

"But her end is bitter as wormwood, sharp as a two-edged sword."

Proverbs 5:4

"He hath filled me with bitterness, he hath made me drunken with wormwood."

Lamentations 3:15

The wormwood bush is mentioned several times in the Bible and New Testament as a metaphor for bitterness, torment and grief; small wonder, since it has an extremely bitter taste that lingers in the mouth for a long time. Several types of wormwood grow in the Holy Land and around the world, and they all have medicinal and other interesting properties.

141

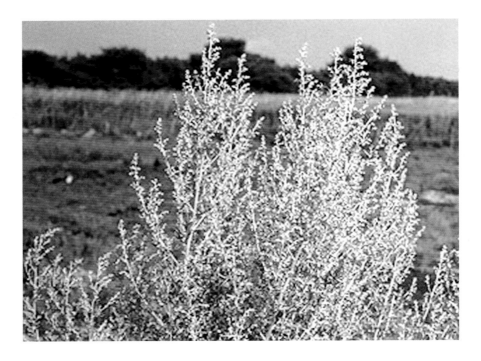

The type of wormwood most likely to be the one mentioned in the Bible is the white wormwood, a low bush about a foot and a half high that grows in the desert. It has large leaves in winter and tiny ones in summer, and between August and October, small, pale yellow flowers bloom at the tip of its slender branches. The plant is covered in fine hairs that contain oils with a powerful scent. Another type, the Judean wormwood, is similar in height and coloration, although it is a larger bush with paler leaves. A third type, the Artemisia absinatum, is taller – two to four feet high – and blooms in May and June.

The properties of wormwood were known as early as 1600 BCE, when the ancient Egyptians used it to rid the body of parasites. According to legend, it was left in the serpent's wake as he slithered out of the Garden of Eden. An even more interesting fact about this plant is that the larger species mentioned above, Artemisia absinatum, is used to produce the infamous alcoholic beverage, absinthe. In fact, it is mentioned in the Talmud, and it is said that in Biblical times, mixing the bitter juice of the wormwood plant with wine made for quite a popular cocktail…

Various types of wormwood are used in a range of natural remedies. The above-mentioned white wormwood is dubbed the "king of herbs" by the Bedouin in the Negev Desert, since it is used to treat a dozen problems ranging from stomach-aches to snake bites. A small stalk of white wormwood in a cup of warm tea is good for an upset stomach. For stomach poisoning – particularly in children – as well as for coughs and fevers, a handful of wormwood leaves is cooked in a glass of olive oil for half an hour. The oil is filtered, and the dosage is a spoonful every morning.

A handful of wormwood leaves cooked in four ounces of butter, then filtered, is effective for treating colds and other respiratory illnesses. Three spoonfuls a day do the trick. The same handful of leaves can be cooked in plain water, and the filtrate applied to eye infections.

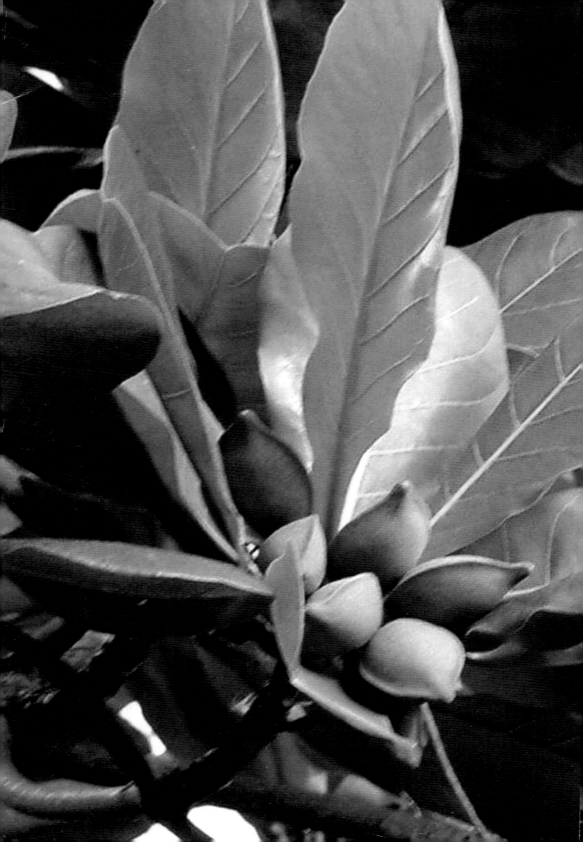